INTEGRATING SOCIAL CARE INTO THE DELIVERY OF HEALTH CARE

MOVING UPSTREAM TO IMPROVE THE NATION'S HEALT

Committee on Integrating Social Needs Care into the Delivery of Health Care to Improve the Nation's Health

Board on Health Care Services

Health and Medicine Division

A Consensus Study Report of

The National Academies of
SCIENCES · ENGINEERING · MEDICINE

THE NATIONAL ACADEMIES PRESS
Washington, DC
www.nap.edu

THE NATIONAL ACADEMIES PRESS 500 Fifth Street, NW Washington, DC 20001

This activity was supported by agreements between the National Academy of Sciences and Archstone Foundation; Association of Oncology Social Work; Bader Philanthropies; Chicago Community Trust; Community Memorial Foundation; Council on Social Work Education; Episcopal Health Foundation; Health Foundation of Western and Central New York; Healthy Communities Foundation; Helen Rehr Center for Social Work Practice; Josiah Macy Jr. Foundation; Kaiser Permanente National Community Benefit; National Association of Social Workers (NASW) and NASW Foundation; New York Community Trust; Robert Wood Johnson Foundation; SCAN Foundation; and Society for Social Work Leadership in Health Care.

Additional support was obtained from the Boston University Center for Innovation in Social Work and Health social work academic program match campaign. Contributing academic programs were Adelphi University School of Social Work; Baylor University Diana R. Garland School of Social Work; Binghamton University SUNY College of Community and Public Affairs Department of Social Work; Boston College School of Social Work; Brown School at Washington University in St. Louis; California Association of Deans and Directors of Social Work Programs; Case Western Reserve University Jack, Joseph, and Morton Mandel School of Applied Social Sciences; Clark Atlanta University Whitney M. Young, Jr., School of Social Work; Colorado State University–Pueblo Department of Social Work; Colorado State University School of Social Work; Columbia University School of Social Work; Erikson Institute Graduate School in Child Development; Fordham University Graduate School of Social Service; Georgia State University School of Social Work; Howard University School of Social Work; Long Island University Social Work, Brooklyn and Post campuses; Loyola University Chicago School of Social Work; Monmouth University School of Social Work; New York State Association of Deans and Directors of Schools of Social Work; New York University Silver School of Social Work; North Carolina State University School of Social Work; Portland State University School of Social Work; Rutgers University School of Social Work; Saint Louis University School of Social Work; Salem State University School of Social Work; San Diego State University School of Social Work; Simmons University School of Social Work; Smith College School for Social Work; Springfield College School of Social Work; St. Louis Group for Excellence in Social Work Research and Education; Stephen F. Austin State University School of School Work; SUNY Stony Brook School of Social Welfare; The Ohio State University College of Social Work; The University of Alabama School of Social Work; The University of Chicago School of Social Service Administration and Center for Health Administration Studies; The University of Southern Mississippi School of Social Work; The University of Texas at Arlington School of Social Work; The University of Utah College of Social Work; University at Albany SUNY School of Social Welfare; University at Buffalo SUNY School of Social Work; University of California, Berkeley, School of Social Welfare; University of California, Los Angeles, Luskin School of Public Affairs Department of Social Welfare; University of Cincinnati School of Social Work; University of Connecticut

School of Social Work; University of Georgia School of Social Work; University of Hawaii at Manoa Myron B. Thompson School of Social Work; University of Houston Graduate College of Social Work; University of Illinois at Chicago Jane Addams College of Social Work; University of Kentucky College of Social Work; University of Louisville Kent School of Social Work; University of Maryland School of Social Work; University of Michigan School of Social Work; University of Missouri School of Social Work; University of North Carolina at Chapel Hill School of Social Work; University of North Carolina at Charlotte School of Social Work; University of Oklahoma Anne and Henry Zarrow School of Social Work and Center for Social Work in Healthcare; University of Pittsburgh School of Social Work; University of South Carolina College of Social Work; University of South Florida School of Social Work; University of Southern California Suzanne Dworak–Peck School of Social Work; University of Washington School of Social Work; University of Wisconsin–Milwaukee Helen Bader School of Social Welfare; University of Wisconsin–Whitewater Department of Social Work; and Westfield State University Department of Social Work. Any opinions, findings, conclusions, or recommendations expressed in this publication do not necessarily reflect the views of any organization or agency that provided support for the project.

International Standard Book Number-13: 978-0-309-49343-7
International Standard Book Number-10: 0-309-49343-9
Digital Object Identifier: https://doi.org/10.17226/25467
Library of Congress Control Number: 2019951417

Additional copies of this publication are available from the National Academies Press, 500 Fifth Street, NW, Keck 360, Washington, DC 20001; (800) 624-6242 or (202) 334-3313; http://www.nap.edu.

Printed in the United States of America

Suggested citation: National Academies of Sciences, Engineering, and Medicine. 2019. *Integrating social care into the delivery of health care: Moving upstream to improve the nation's health.* Washington, DC: The National Academies Press. https://doi.org/10.17226/25467.

The National Academies of
SCIENCES • ENGINEERING • MEDICINE

The **National Academy of Sciences** was established in 1863 by an Act of Congress, signed by President Lincoln, as a private, nongovernmental institution to advise the nation on issues related to science and technology. Members are elected by their peers for outstanding contributions to research. Dr. Marcia McNutt is president.

The **National Academy of Engineering** was established in 1964 under the charter of the National Academy of Sciences to bring the practices of engineering to advising the nation. Members are elected by their peers for extraordinary contributions to engineering. Dr. John L. Anderson is president.

The **National Academy of Medicine** (formerly the Institute of Medicine) was established in 1970 under the charter of the National Academy of Sciences to advise the nation on medical and health issues. Members are elected by their peers for distinguished contributions to medicine and health. Dr. Victor J. Dzau is president.

The three Academies work together as the **National Academies of Sciences, Engineering, and Medicine** to provide independent, objective analysis and advice to the nation and conduct other activities to solve complex problems and inform public policy decisions. The National Academies also encourage education and research, recognize outstanding contributions to knowledge, and increase public understanding in matters of science, engineering, and medicine.

Learn more about the National Academies of Sciences, Engineering, and Medicine at **www.nationalacademies.org.**

The National Academies of

SCIENCES · ENGINEERING · MEDICINE

Consensus Study Reports published by the National Academies of Sciences, Engineering, and Medicine document the evidence-based consensus on the study's statement of task by an authoring committee of experts. Reports typically include findings, conclusions, and recommendations based on information gathered by the committee and the committee's deliberations. Each report has been subjected to a rigorous and independent peer-review process and it represents the position of the National Academies on the statement of task.

Proceedings published by the National Academies of Sciences, Engineering, and Medicine chronicle the presentations and discussions at a workshop, symposium, or other event convened by the National Academies. The statements and opinions contained in proceedings are those of the participants and are not endorsed by other participants, the planning committee, or the National Academies.

For information about other products and activities of the National Academies, please visit www.nationalacademies.org/about/whatwedo.

COMMITTEE ON INTEGRATING SOCIAL NEEDS CARE INTO THE DELIVERY OF HEALTH CARE TO IMPROVE THE NATION'S HEALTH

KIRSTEN BIBBINS-DOMINGO (*Chair*), Lee Goldman, M.D., Endowed Chair in Medicine; Professor and Chair, Department of Epidemiology and Biostatistics, University of California, San Francisco

TOYIN AJAYI, Chief Health Officer, Cityblock Health

TAMARA CADET, Associate Professor, School of Social Work, Simmons University

LISA A. COOPER, Bloomberg Distinguished Professor, James F. Fries Professor of Medicine, Director, Johns Hopkins Center for Health Equity, Johns Hopkins University School of Medicine and Bloomberg School of Public Health

KAREN DeSALVO, Professor of Medicine, The University of Texas at Austin, Dell Medical School

CHRIS ESGUERRA, Senior Medical Director, Blue Shield of California

JANET C. FRANK, Adjunct Associate Professor, Faculty Associate, University of California, Los Angeles (UCLA) Center for Health Policy Research, UCLA Fielding School of Public Health

RACHEL GOLD, Senior Investigator, Kaiser Permanente Northwest Center for Health Research and Lead Research Scientist, OCHIN

ROBYN GOLDEN, Associate Vice President, Population Health and Aging, Rush University Medical Center

LAURA GOTTLIEB, Director, Social Interventions Research and Evaluation Network, Department of Family and Community Medicine, University of California, San Francisco

SEAN JOE, Benjamin E. Youngdhal Professor of Social Development, Brown School, Washington University in Saint Louis

CHRISTOPHER KOLLER, President, Milbank Memorial Fund

CINDY MANN, Partner, Manatt, Phelps & Phillips, LLP

DIANA J. MASON, Senior Policy Service Professor, Center for Health Policy and Media Engagement, School of Nursing, The George Washington University

KEDAR MATE, Chief Innovation and Education Officer, Institute for Healthcare Improvement

EDWARD SALSBERG, Director of Health Workforce Studies, Health Workforce Institute, The George Washington University

ELIZABETH CUERVO TILSON, State Health Director and Chief Medical Officer, North Carolina Department of Health and Human Services
KEEGAN WARREN-CLEM, Director, Austin Medical–Legal Partnership, Texas Legal Services Center and People's Community Clinic

Study Staff

ABIGAIL MITCHELL, Study Director
MEGAN KEARNEY, Associate Program Officer
ANNALEE GONZALES, Administrative Assistant
MICAH WINOGRAD, Financial Officer
SHARYL NASS, Director, Board on Health Care Services

Consultants

AMBER HALEY, Health Policy and Management, Gillings School of Global Public Health, University of North Carolina at Chapel Hill
ALLISON MYERS, Director, Oregon State University Center for Health Innovation

Editorial Consultant

ROBERT POOL

Reviewers

This Consensus Study Report was reviewed in draft form by individuals chosen for their diverse perspectives and technical expertise. The purpose of this independent review is to provide candid and critical comments that will assist the National Academies of Sciences, Engineering, and Medicine in making each published report as sound as possible and to ensure that it meets the institutional standards for quality, objectivity, evidence, and responsiveness to the study charge. The review comments and draft manuscript remain confidential to protect the integrity of the deliberative process.

We thank the following individuals for their review of this report:

JEFFERY BRENNER, UnitedHealthcare
KARINA W. DAVISON, Northwell Health
KAREN DONELAN, Health Policy Research Center at the Mongan Institute, Harvard Medical School
ERIN P. FRAHER, University of North Carolina at Chapel Hill School of Medicine
LAURAN HARDIN, National Center for Complex Health and Social Needs, Camden Coalition
PETER MARAMALDI, Simmons School of Social Work and Harvard T.H. Chan School of Public Health
HEATHER A. McCABE, Indiana University School of Social Work
VICTORIA M. RIZZO, University at Albany State University of New York School of Social Welfare

NIRAV R. SHAH, Stanford University
KATHERINE SWARTZ, Harvard T.H. Chan School of Public Health
ELLEN-MARIE WHELAN, Centers for Medicare & Medicaid Services

Although the reviewers listed above provided many constructive comments and suggestions, they were not asked to endorse the conclusions or recommendations of this report, nor did they see the final draft before its release. The review of this report was overseen by **SUSAN CURRY,** The University of Iowa, and **BRADFORD H. GRAY,** Urban Institute. They were responsible for making certain that an independent examination of this report was carried out in accordance with the standards of the National Academies and that all review comments were carefully considered. Responsibility for the final content rests entirely with the authoring committee and the National Academies.

Acknowledgments

We, the members of the National Academies of Sciences, Engineering, and Medicine's Committee on Integrating Social Needs Care into the Delivery of Health Care to Improve the Nation's Health, wish to express our sincere gratitude to the many individuals and groups who helped with this report.

Our work would not have been possible without the generosity of the sponsors. We would like to thank Archstone Foundation; Association of Oncology Social Work; Bader Philanthropies; Chicago Community Trust; Community Memorial Foundation; Council on Social Work Education; Episcopal Health Foundation; Health Foundation of Western and Central New York; Healthy Communities Foundation; Helen Rehr Center for Social Work Practice; Josiah Macy Jr. Foundation; Kaiser Permanente National Community Benefit; National Association of Social Workers (NASW) and NASW Foundation; New York Community Trust; Robert Wood Johnson Foundation; SCAN Foundation; and Society for Social Work Leadership in Health Care. We also would like to thank the social work academic programs that contributed to this work through a match campaign sponsored by the Boston University Center for Innovation in Social Work and Health:

Adelphi University School of Social Work
Baylor University Diana R. Garland School of Social Work
Binghamton University SUNY College of Community and Public Affairs Department of Social Work
Boston College School of Social Work
Brown School at Washington University in St. Louis

California Association of Deans and Directors of Social Work Programs
Case Western Reserve University Jack, Joseph, and Morton Mandel School of Applied Social Sciences
Clark Atlanta University Whitney M. Young, Jr., School of Social Work
Colorado State University–Pueblo Department of Social Work
Colorado State University School of Social Work
Columbia University School of Social Work
Erikson Institute Graduate School in Child Development
Fordham University Graduate School of Social Service
Georgia State University School of Social Work
Howard University School of Social Work
Long Island University Social Work, Brooklyn and Post campuses
Loyola University Chicago School of Social Work
Monmouth University School of Social Work
New York State Association of Deans and Directors of Schools of Social Work
New York University Silver School of Social Work
North Carolina State University School of Social Work
Portland State University School of Social Work
Rutgers University School of Social Work
Saint Louis University School of Social Work
Salem State University School of Social Work
San Diego State University School of Social Work
Simmons University School of Social Work
Smith College School for Social Work
Springfield College School of Social Work
St. Louis Group for Excellence in Social Work Research and Education
Stephen F. Austin State University School of School Work
SUNY Stony Brook School of Social Welfare
The Ohio State University College of Social Work
The University of Alabama School of Social Work
The University of Chicago School of Social Service Administration and Center for Health Administration Studies
The University of Southern Mississippi School of Social Work
The University of Texas at Arlington School of Social Work
The University of Utah College of Social Work
University at Albany SUNY School of Social Welfare
University at Buffalo SUNY School of Social Work
University of California, Berkeley, School of Social Welfare

University of California, Los Angeles, Luskin School of Public Affairs Department of Social Welfare
University of Cincinnati School of Social Work
University of Connecticut School of Social Work
University of Georgia School of Social Work
University of Hawaii at Manoa Myron B. Thompson School of Social Work
University of Houston Graduate College of Social Work
University of Illinois at Chicago Jane Addams College of Social Work
University of Kentucky College of Social Work
University of Louisville Kent School of Social Work
University of Maryland School of Social Work
University of Michigan School of Social Work
University of Missouri School of Social Work
University of North Carolina at Chapel Hill School of Social Work
University of North Carolina at Charlotte School of Social Work
University of Oklahoma Anne and Henry Zarrow School of Social Work and Center for Social Work in Healthcare
University of Pittsburgh School of Social Work
University of South Carolina College of Social Work
University of South Florida School of Social Work
University of Southern California Suzanne Dworak–Peck School of Social Work
University of Washington School of Social Work
University of Wisconsin–Milwaukee Helen Bader School of Social Welfare
University of Wisconsin–Whitewater Department of Social Work
Westfield State University Department of Social Work

We are grateful to the Gordon and Betty Moore Foundation and to the National Academy of Medicine's Culture of Health Program for providing financial support for report dissemination and communications efforts.

Over the course of the study, we received valuable information and insight from a number of individuals with expertise in fields related to health-related social care. Thank you to the presenters at our public meetings:

Sara Bachman, Boston University School of Social Work
Michelle Brazeal, Mississippi Integrated Health and Disaster Program and The University of Southern Mississippi
Darla Spence Coffey, Council on Social Work Education

Kelly Craig, Camden Coalition of Healthcare Providers
Jolene Fassbinder, Archstone Foundation
Kathryn Haslanger, JASA
Reverend Debra Hickman, Sisters Together and Reaching, Inc.
Kristie Kulinski, Administration for Community Living, U.S. Department of Health and Human Services
Natasha Lifton, New York Community Trust
Angelo McClain, National Association of Social Workers
Susan Mende, Robert Wood Johnson Foundation
Tim Rehner, School of Social Work, The University of Southern Mississippi
Susan Reinhard, AARP Public Policy Institute
Victoria M. Rizzo, School of Social Welfare, University at Albany SUNY
Walter Rosenberg, Social Work and Community Health, Rush University Medical Center
Loel Solomon, Kaiser Permanente National Community Benefit
Laura Taylor, Veterans Health Administration, U.S. Department of Veterans Affairs
Roberta Waite, College of Nursing and Health Professions, Drexel University and Stephen and Sandra Sheller 11th Street Family Health Service
Michelle M. Washko, National Center for Health Workforce Analysis, Health Resources and Services Administration, U.S. Department of Health and Human Services
Randi Woods, Sisters Together and Reaching, Inc.

We also thank Dave Chokshi, NYC Health + Hospitals, and Louise Cohen and Riley Moreen, Primary Care Development Corporation, for providing information to the committee at its request.

We appreciate the considerable efforts of Bonnie Ewald, Rush University Medical Center, and of the Social Work in Health Care Leadership Workgroup convened by the Center for Health and Social Care Integration, who were instrumental in conceiving the idea for the study and working to move it forward. In addition to the study staff, we would like to thank National Academies' staff members Daniel Bearss[1] and Jorge Mendoza-Torres for their research assistance, Kyra Cappelucci and Greta Gorman for their oversight of report communications efforts, and Karen Helsing for her assistance with fundraising for the study.

[1] Daniel Bearss passed away on July 5, 2019. A senior librarian at the National Academies since 2005, his assistance with literature searches and other research for this report was invaluable.

Contents

Summary

The consistent and compelling evidence concerning how social determinants shape health has led to a growing recognition throughout the health care sector that improvements in overall health metrics are likely to depend—at least in part—on attention being paid to these social determinants. The shift in the health care sector toward value-based payments that incentivize prevention and improved health and health care outcomes for persons and populations rather than service delivery alone has made possible expanded approaches to addressing health-related factors that may be upstream from the clinical encounter. And there is increasing interest in the role of the health care sector in mitigating adverse social determinants (termed "social risk factors" and including a lack of access to stable housing, nutritious food, or reliable transportation) in order to achieve more equitable health outcomes. The combined result of these trends has been a growing emphasis on health care systems paying attention to upstream factors and addressing the social determinants of health (SDOH).[1] Taking social risk factors into account is critical to improving both primary prevention and the treatment of acute and chronic illness because social contexts influence the delivery and outcomes of health care.

In considering how health care systems should address these social determinants, a number of important questions arise, including how to integrate social care (that is, services that address health-related social risk factors and social needs) into clinical practice and what kinds of

[1] A list of social determinants of health is included in Table 1-1 of this report.

infrastructure will be required to facilitate such activities. To begin addressing these questions, a broad coalition of foundations, social work associations, educational institutions, and other organizations came together to support this National Academies of Sciences, Engineering, and Medicine (the National Academies) study. The study was intended to examine the potential for integrating services addressing social needs and the SDOH into the delivery of health care with the ultimate goal of achieving better health outcomes.[2] The National Academies appointed a committee of 18 subject-matter experts to address this task. Specifically, the committee was asked to assess several factors: the approaches to social care integration that are currently being taken by health care providers and systems as well as any new or emerging approaches and opportunities; the current roles in such integration that are being taken on by different disciplines and organizations as well as new or emerging roles and types of providers; and the current and emerging efforts to design health care systems in such a way as to improve the nation's health and reduces health inequities. The committee also was asked to recommend how to expand social care services, to better coordinate roles for social care providers in interprofessional care teams in diverse health settings, and to optimize the effectiveness of social care services to improve health and health care.

Over the course of the 18-month study, the committee held four in-person meetings and two Web-based meetings to gather evidence, review and deliberate on the evidence, and develop conclusions and recommendations. Several types of evidence were considered, including peer-reviewed literature, reports from governmental agencies and private organizations, books, websites, and invited presentations to the committee during public sessions. Although the committee cast a wide net in its efforts to identify relevant sources of information, it did not conduct a systematic literature review. As part of the National Academies consensus study process, the committee's draft report underwent a rigorous, independent external review by another group of experts to ensure that the report addressed its charge, that its findings are supported by the scientific evidence, that its exposition and organization are effective, and that it is impartial and objective.

FIVE HEALTH CARE ACTIVITIES TO BETTER INTEGRATE SOCIAL CARE

The committee identified five complementary activities that can facilitate the integration of social care into health care. The activities are

[2] The complete Statement of Task is presented in Chapter 1 of this report.

awareness, adjustment, assistance, alignment, and advocacy (see Figure S-1 and Table S-1). The specific types of activities that are undertaken will likely vary across health care settings and within settings and also by the social factors being addressed, and the context of a setting will influence which specific types of social and health care integration activities are adopted.

Some health care systems have had success using these five types of activities to strengthen social care services and to link social care with improved health outcomes. However, in most cases where social care activities occur, there have been few robust outcome evaluations carried out, which limited the committee's ability to make recommendations about specific evidence-based practices. Rather, the committee focused on a framework that describes the scope of these practices.

FINDINGS

Each of the five activities described in the previous section—awareness, adjustment, assistance, alignment, and advocacy—involves systems-level changes. After a review of the evidence base on existing and emerging activities and opportunities for integrating social care into health care, the committee identified three key necessities for successful integration: an appropriately staffed and trained workforce, health information technology innovations, and new financing models.

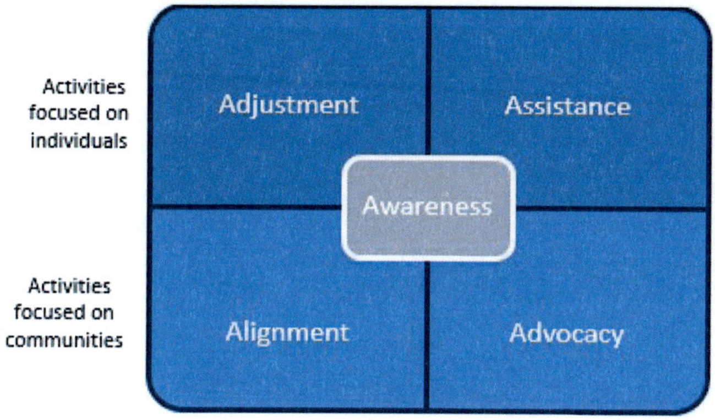

FIGURE S-1 Health care system activities that strengthen social care integration.

TABLE S-1
Definitions of Health Care System Activities That Strengthen Social Care Integration

Activity	Definition	Transportation-Related Example
Awareness	Activities that identify the social risks and assets of defined patients and populations.	Ask people about their access to transportation.
Adjustment	Activities that focus on altering clinical care to accommodate identified social barriers.	Reduce the need for in-person health care appointments by using other options such as telehealth appointments.
Assistance	Activities that reduce social risk by providing assistance in connecting patients with relevant social care resources.	Provide transportation vouchers so that patients can travel to health care appointments. Vouchers can be used for ride-sharing services or public transit.
Alignment	Activities undertaken by health care systems to understand existing social care assets in the community, organize them to facilitate synergies, and invest in and deploy them to positively affect health outcomes.	Invest in community ride-sharing or time-bank programs.
Advocacy	Activities in which health care organizations work with partner social care organizations to promote policies that facilitate the creation and redeployment of assets or resources to address health and social needs.	Work to promote policies that fundamentally change the transportation infrastructure within the community.

Workforce

All members of an interprofessional team working to address health-related social needs may have a role in carrying out awareness, adjustment, assistance, alignment, and advocacy activities. The social care workers on the team may include nurses; physicians; social workers; community health workers; social service navigators, aides, assistants, and trained volunteers; home health aides; personal care aides; family caregivers; case managers; gerontologists; lawyers; and others. The committee found that

- Effectively integrating social care into the delivery of health care requires effective interprofessional teams that include experts in social care.
- The social care workforce can include many types of workers. Social workers are specialists in providing social care who have a long history of working within health care delivery. Models

that include community health workers show promise. As models continue to evolve and develop, roles may expand for other workers, such as social service navigators, aides, and assistants; trained volunteers; home health aides and personal care aides; and family caregivers. Other fields are emerging to meet the social needs of older adults (e.g., gerontology) and other specific populations. Integrating other professions—such as lawyers through medical–legal partnerships—also holds promise.

- Understanding the role each member of an interprofessional team plays in the awareness, adjustment, assistance, alignment, and advocacy activities is important for ensuring effective collaboration among team members and for maximizing their ability to address patients' social needs.
- In order to effectively address social care in the delivery of health care, interprofessional team members should operate at their full scope of practice. Federal, state, and institutional barriers limit the scope of practice and the full use of social workers and other social care workers in caring for patients, such as in providing care management as part of an interprofessional team.
- For interprofessional teams to effectively address social care in the context of health care financing structures need to be aligned. Federal, state, and institutional barriers exist that may limit the adequate payment of social workers, gerontologists, and other social care workers.
- Research is needed on workforce issues related to integrating social care and health care, including studying the effect on health and financial outcomes of various configurations of the health care workforce intended to better address the social needs of the populations served.

Data and Digital Tools

Advances in technology that allow for the application of data and digital tools have the potential to improve efforts by health care systems and their social care partners to address health-related social needs via awareness, adjustment, assistance, alignment, and advocacy activities. Many sources of data exist, including health care claims, electronic health records, census data, and community-level findings concerning the SDOH. The types of digital tools available include predictive analytics, natural language processing, geocoding and hotspotting (the strategic use of data to reallocate resources to a small subset of high-needs, high-cost patients), point-of-care decision support, augmented intelligence, the Internet of Things, telehealth and other virtual care, automated interactions (e.g., chat bots and holograms), self-driving cars, and digital platforms for interoperability. The committee found that

- Data and technology have transformed the consumer experience in many sectors of life and are doing so in health care.
- Billions of dollars in federal resources spurred the digitization of health care through the widespread adoption of electronic health records and interoperability. Social care has not benefited from the same resources and policy attention as has the health care sector, and it lags far behind in digitization.
- Private equity has supported the health technology economy. Venture capitalists are increasingly investing in health technology startup companies that are working to address the SDOH.
- Local efforts to share health care and social care data exist, including emerging private-sector solutions. These are not supported by a strategic national vision or coupled with resources or defined technology standards.
- Interoperability and data sharing between health care and social care are hampered by the lack of infrastructure, data standards, and modern technology architecture shared between and among organizations.
- With an increasing number of stakeholders sharing protected health information in order to coordinate care, data privacy and security remain challenging elements to manage.
- Digital approaches to integrating social care into health care may increase existing health disparities by exacerbating the digital divide and by codifying bias within health systems.
- There is a paucity of rigorous research that can inform a collective understanding of best practices and outcomes of efforts to integrate social care with health care.

Financing

The financing of health care offers an opportunity to better integrate social care into health care, but substantial barriers exist to doing so. The key challenges identified by the committee are how the legal definition of health care affects the inclusion of social care, how methods for paying providers incentivize or disincentivize the integration of social care into health care delivery, how quality and accountability for the integration of social care are defined and measured, how care for populations with complex social and health needs is financed, and the limited administrative capacity of many social care providers. The committee grouped its findings into the following categories:

- *Definition of health care and how it affects the inclusion of social care as part of health care*
  - o Statute and contract definitions of what constitutes health care have been largely driven by the cultural history of medicine and have made it less likely that social care activities would be included in the health care setting.
  - o Within existing definitions of health care, state Medicaid programs and their contracted managed care plans and accountable providers are innovating with awareness, adjustment, assistance, and alignment activities to pay for social care in health care settings using state plan amendment authority and the waiver process.
  - o There remains great variation among states in the level of social care activity; the Centers for Medicare & Medicaid Services (CMS) provides only limited guidance about permissible social care activities and benefits.
  - o Rate-setting processes for health plans and providers can be influential in obtaining financing for the integration of social care in the health care setting; the key factors are the rates calculated, risk adjustment elements to those rates, performance incentives, and the definition of medical services and quality improvement activities in the calculation of medical loss ratios.
  - o Among the states with approved waivers there is much experimentation, with informal mechanisms for learning the results of the experimentation. Formal evaluations of these waiver activities typically are not timely and do not influence policy and practice.
  - o The Medicare Advantage plan bidding process insufficiently promotes competition on the basis of care coordination and high-quality care.
  - o Medicare's new supplemental benefits guidance to Medicare Advantage plans, made possible by the Creating High-Quality Results and Outcomes Necessary to Improve Chronic Care Act of 2018 (CHRONIC Care Act),[3] has created new opportunities to integrate social care into the health care of Medicare beneficiaries.
- *Incentives to integrate health care and social care*
  - o The prevailing model of health care provider payment—fee-for-service—does not encourage the integration of social care. The current shift to alternate payment models led by the

[3] Section III of Public Law 115-123, February 9, 2018.

Center for Medicare & Medicaid Innovation (a center within CMS) activities—particularly the shift to accountable care organizations—aligns incentives for the provision of social care.

- Just as state Medicaid programs are experimenting with different covered services definitions, they are innovating with new methods to pay providers, such as through accountable care organizations, in part to encourage more social care integration work. There is less such work taking place for commercial and Medicare populations. Furthermore, great variation among states exists in the types of population-based payment models (i.e., models in which a provider agrees to accept responsibility for the health of a group of patients in exchange for a set amount of money) that are being deployed, and, as with covered service definitions, states and, in some cases, their contracted health plans are not performing formal evaluation of these activities.

- *Quality and accountability*
  - Definitions of health care services and conditions have historically provided insufficient clarity and guidance for integrating and addressing social care.
  - Population outcome measures for accountable entities, or accountable care organizations, are numerous and highly variable among the states.
  - The conclusions included in a previous National Academies report on adjusting Medicare payments for social risk factors[4] have not been applied in Medicaid settings to payments or outcome measures.
  - Even with good accountability measures, health plans and providers struggle to justify investments when returns are delayed and accrue to collaborators. The lack of continuous eligibility for Medicaid benefits exacerbates this problem, as does the long-term nature of the returns on investments in social care integration and on upstream investment in pediatric populations. Geographic exclusivity, which limits the number of providers operating within a region, makes it possible for partners to make longer-term investments, but this is not possible in populous settings.

[4] National Academies of Sciences, Engineering, and Medicine. 2017. *Accounting for social risk factors in Medicare payment*. Washington, DC: The National Academies Press. https://doi.org/10.17226/23635.

  - The Internal Revenue Service (IRS) community benefit standard is another opportunity to finance the integration of social care in health care settings. Experience has shown varying levels of engagement by health systems, little enforcement by the IRS, and varying levels of aligned attention from states and communities.
- *Financing care for patients with complex health and social needs*
  - Patients enrolled in both Medicaid and Medicare have the highest social needs, but the division of their health care financing between state and federal agencies creates barriers to addressing those needs in a way that integrates social care.
  - The Programs of All-Inclusive Care for the Elderly program enrolls a fraction of dual eligibles and has demonstrated mixed results.
  - No systematic evaluations exist for dual-eligible special needs programs in part because each state's program is unique. The CHRONIC Care Act mandated the evaluation of dual-eligible special needs programs, which may assist with standardization.
  - The financial alignment demonstration for dual eligibles shows that while care innovation increases with alignment, administrative and financial challenges remain.
  - Evaluations of the financial alignment demonstration have found savings in two states and improved health care use outcomes in additional states. The demonstration has been extended and expanded to accrue more of the data needed to evaluate its effectiveness.
- *Capacity building for social care providers*
  - Social service agencies and health care organizations have historically not worked together, and they are funded by different systems.
  - Health systems may "medicalize" the integration of social care into health care. Health systems often use models of care requiring research, diagnostic codes, and technical specialization, which adds cost and complexity, with the ultimate result being effects on population health that are neutral or negative.
  - The administrative costs of social care providers could increase as a result of efforts to integrate social care into a health care setting based on a medical model for consultation and referral.

RECOMMENDATIONS

Enabling the health care sector to engage in activities that strengthen social care and community resources will require new approaches to system design, staffing, information and technology systems, financing, and research. The committee identified five goals whose accomplishment will result in better integration of social care into health care, which may in turn result in improved health and reduced health disparities. Those goals are to

1. Design health care delivery to integrate social care into health care, guided by the five health care system activities—awareness, adjustment, assistance, alignment, and advocacy.
2. Build a workforce to integrate social care into health care delivery.
3. Develop a digital infrastructure that is interoperable between health care and social care organizations.
4. Finance the integration of health care and social care.
5. Fund, conduct, and translate research and evaluation on the effectiveness and implementation of social care practices in health care settings.

Goal 1. Design health care delivery to integrate social care into health care.

Recommendation 1. Health care organizations should take steps to integrate social care into health care. Specific steps include

a. Make and communicate an organizational commitment to addressing health-related social needs and health disparities at the community and individual levels.
b. Recognize that comprehensive health care should include understanding an individual's social context. Evidence is rapidly accumulating concerning the most effective strategies for screening and assessing for social risk factors and social needs. Such strategies should include standardized and validated questions, as available, and should use interoperable data systems to document results.
c. Use patient-centered care[5] models to more routinely incorporate social risk data into care decisions.

[5] *Patient-centered care* is defined as providing care that is respectful of and responsive to individual patient preferences, needs, and values, and ensuring that patient values guide all clinical decisions (Institute of Medicine. 2001. *Crossing the quality chasm: A new health system for the 21st century*. Washington, DC: National Academy Press. https://doi.org/10.17226/10027).

d. Design and implement integrated care systems using approaches that engage patients, community partners, frontline staff, social care workers, and clinicians in planning and evaluation and that incorporate the preferences of patients and communities.
e. Include social care workers as being integral to a team-based approach to designing and delivering health care.
f. Establish linkages and communication pathways between health care and social service providers. This is important for personal care aides, home care aides, and others who provide care and support for seriously ill and disabled patients and who have extensive knowledge of patients' social needs.
g. Develop and finance referral relationships with selected social care providers when feasible, supported by operational integration such as co-location or patient information systems. Social care providers and health care providers should establish a formal understanding and accountability within their contracting and referral relationships.
h. Support the development of those infrastructure components needed to meet the goal of care integration, including the redesign and refinement of workflows, technical assistance and support, staff with the ability to support the redesign, champions of the redesign, information on best practices, health information technology to enhance integration, and support for community partners and their infrastructure needs.

Goal 2. Build a workforce to integrate social care into health care delivery.

Recommendation 2a. State legislatures, licensing boards, professional associations, and federal agencies should develop, expand, and standardize the scopes of practice of social workers, community health workers, gerontologists, and other social care workers.

Recommendation 2b. Social workers and other social care workers should be considered to be providers who are eligible for reimbursement by payers. Public and private payers should create standards for the reimbursement of social care, including assessment and such treatment as chronic care management, behavioral health integration, and transitional care management. Medicare/Medicaid payment advisory commissions should evaluate models in which social workers and other social care workers are reimbursement-eligible providers of social care services.

Recommendation 2c. Funders of health care workforce training (e.g., the U.S. Department of Health and Human Services, the U.S. Department of Veterans Affairs, and foundations) should include the social care workforce in their education, training, and practice initiatives.

Recommendation 2d. Schools for health professions (including schools of medicine and nursing) as well as continuing education programs should incorporate competency-based curricula on social care. Curricula should include evidence on the social determinants of health, protocols for working in interprofessional teams to address social needs in health care settings, interpersonal and organizational approaches to advancing health equity and decreasing health disparities, and competencies relating to collecting, securing, and using data and technology to facilitate social and health care integration. Schools of health professions should also engage social workers in instructional roles in order to model their participation in interprofessional teams and to provide information on social risk screening and social care resources and referrals.

Recommendation 2e. Credentialing organizations for medicine, nursing, and other health professions should incorporate knowledge about the social determinants of health and the importance of addressing social needs in licensing examinations and continuing education requirements.

Recommendation 2f. Schools of social work as well as continuing education programs should use competency-based curricula on social care. In addition to educating students about the social determinants of health and health disparities, the curricula should include information about effective models that integrate social care and health care delivery, the interprofessional workforce, technology, and payment models that facilitate implementation and competencies relating to collecting, securing, and using data and technology to facilitate social and health care integration.

Recommendation 2g. State agencies and academic institutions, including community colleges, should develop standards for training and advancement (e.g., career ladder programs) for community health workers and other emerging social care workers.

Recommendation 2h. Foundations and other funders should commission a follow-up comprehensive report on the role of social work in health care as social care and health care integration continues to evolve.

Recommendation 2i. Foundations and other funders should fund a campaign to raise awareness among the health care professions and others about the value and contributions of social workers and other social care workers in health care.

Goal 3. Develop a digital infrastructure that is interoperable between health care and social care organizations.

Recommendation 3a. The federal government should establish a 21st-century social care digital infrastructure on a scale similar to that described in the Health Information and Technology for Economic and Clinical Health Act of 2009,[6] and it should identify and deploy policies and resources to build the internal capacity necessary for social care organizations and consumers to interoperate and interact with each other and the health care system.

Recommendation 3b. The Office of the National Coordinator should be resourced to act on the Patient Protection and Affordable Care Act of 2010[7] Section 1561 recommendations, including the adoption of modern, secure, interoperable digital systems and processes that will allow all partners to share the administrative and other data necessary to enable consumers to seamlessly obtain and maintain the full range of available health care and social care services.

Recommendation 3c. The Office of the National Coordinator should support states and regions as they identify the appropriate interoperable platforms for their communities, based on open standards and a modern technical architecture that supports flexible interfaces to allow the health and social care systems and consumers to share the structured data necessary for care coordination, avoidance of error, and a reduced burden on organizations and people being served.

Recommendation 3d. The Federal Health Information Technology Coordinating Committee should facilitate data sharing at the community level across diverse domains such as health care, housing, and education so as to support social care and health care integration.

Recommendation 3e. Integrating social care and health care requires the sharing of new types of data between new partners, some of whom are covered by the privacy rule promulgated by the Health Insurance Portability and Accountability Act of 1996[8] and some of whom are not; there-

[6] Public Law 111-5, February 17, 2009.
[7] Public Law 111-148, March 23, 2010.
[8] Public Law 104-191, August 21, 1996.

fore, the U.S. Department of Health and Human Services should work with the private sector to disseminate educational tools and guidance on the data security and privacy issues that arise when collecting and sharing personally identifiable information.

Recommendation 3f. The parts of the public and private sectors involved in developing and implementing analytic and technology resources, including cell and Internet access, should do so with an explicit focus on equity; the goal should be to avoid unintended consequences such as perpetuation or aggravation of discrimination and bias and the further marginalization of populations and to proceed with an appreciation of the impact on the existing social care system.

Goal 4. Finance the integration of health care and social care.

Recommendation 4a. The Centers for Medicare & Medicaid Services should clearly define which aspects of social care that Medicaid can pay for as covered services (e.g., in the context of providing care management, targeted case management, and home- and community-based long-term care services and supports as well as within the context of managed care).

Recommendation 4b. State Medicaid agencies should use the flexibility described by the Centers for Medicare & Medicaid Services in the social care that Medicaid pays for as a covered service and make the opportunities and limitations associated with that flexibility clear to health plans and health care and social care service providers.

Recommendation 4c. The Centers for Medicare & Medicaid Services (CMS) should accelerate learning about how the integration of health and social care can improve health and reduce health care costs by encouraging and approving waivers that support social care. Sustainable financing for effective interventions piloted in the waiver should be identified by the state and CMS as an outcome of the waiver.

Recommendation 4d. States should pursue policies of continuous program eligibility to, among other benefits, create stable pools of populations for which entities can be held accountable.

Recommendation 4e. The Centers for Medicare & Medicaid Services should consider additional Medicare reforms that can broaden Medicare coverage rules in a way that is consistent with lessons from Medicaid populations and the Creating High-Quality Results and Outcomes Necessary to Improve Chronic Care Act of 2018 (CHRONIC Care Act).[9] Health plans should take full advantage of the flexibility provided under the CHRONIC Care Act for supplemental benefits under Medicare.

Recommendation 4f. The Centers for Medicare & Medicaid Services and the states should coordinate the coverage and benefits administration of their Medicare and Medicaid dually eligible populations consistent with the emerging lessons of the financial alignment demonstrations. Efforts to improve alignment should be aggressively pursued over the short and long term, with an intentional focus on social care integration.

Recommendation 4g. The Centers for Medicare & Medicaid Services should develop incentives for health care organizations and the managed care programs that contract with Medicaid and Medicare to collaborate with community-based social services, such as area agencies on aging and centers for independent living.

Recommendation 4h. The Centers for Medicare & Medicaid Services, state Medicaid agencies, employers, and health plans should accelerate the movement to alternative payment models. The measurements aimed at assessing value in these models should include activity-based measures for social care integration and outcome measures that reflect social risk and protective factors. These value-based payment and outcome measurement models should incorporate social risk adjustment and stratification in a way that is consistent with previous recommendations from the National Academies of Sciences, Engineering, and Medicine.[10]

Recommendation 4i. The U.S. Department of Health and Human Services, payers, and other private organizations, such as foundations and institutions with community-benefit obligations, should provide funding and technical assistance to support formal contractual relationships between community-based organizations and health care entities.

Recommendation 4j. Federal and state policy makers, health plans, health systems, and private-sector investors should consider collective financing mechanisms to spread risk and create shared returns on investments in social care so that returns do not accrue to a single investor.

---

[9] Public Law 115-123, February 9, 2018.

[10] National Academies of Sciences, Engineering, and Medicine. 2017. *Accounting for social risk factors in Medicare payment*. Washington, DC: The National Academies Press. https://doi.org/10.17226/23635.

Recommendation 4k. Health systems subject to community benefit regulations should comply with those regulations by considering partnering with community organizations to respond to identified community gaps in social care.

Recommendation 4l. States should pursue opportunities to align their hospital licensing requirements and public reporting with federal regulations regarding community benefits to ensure consistent obligations for health systems and to explicitly link their community benefits to the provision of social care.

Goal 5. Fund, conduct, and translate research and evaluation on the effectiveness and implementation of social care practices in health care settings.

Recommendation 5a. Federal and state agencies, payers, providers, delivery systems, and foundations should contribute to advancing research on and the evaluation of the effectiveness and implementation of social care practices.

- The National Institutes of Health (NIH), the Agency for Healthcare Research and Quality (AHRQ), the Centers for Medicare & Medicaid Services (CMS), the Patient-Centered Outcomes Research Institute, the Health Resources and Services Administration (HRSA), and other funders of research and program evaluation should encourage payers, providers, and delivery systems to incorporate a range of study designs and methods that include rapid learning cycles and experimental trials.
- NIH, AHRQ, CMS, foundations, and other funders of research and program evaluation should cultivate and support researchers who have expertise in health services, social sciences, and cross-disciplinary research.
- CMS should fully finance (without state contributions) independent state waiver evaluations to ensure robust evaluation of social care and health care integration pilot programs and to facilitate the dissemination of findings.
- The U.S. Department of Health and Human Services should establish and support a clearinghouse containing information on the best and most promising practices for social care integration in order to provide "lessons learned" to health systems, community-based organizations, researchers, and others.

Recommendation 5b. Funders of health care workforce research (e.g., the Agency for Healthcare Research and Quality and foundations) should include the social care workforce in studies of the effect of the social care workforce on the health and financial outcomes of health care delivery organizations.

Recommendation 5c. The Health Resources and Services Administration and other funders should support studies of the contribution of the social care workforce, including additional workers such as gerontologists and public interest lawyers, to addressing the social determinants of health in health and community care settings.

Recommendation 5d. The Centers for Medicare & Medicaid Services, the U.S. Department of Health and Human Services, state Medicaid agencies, the National Quality Forum, and the National Committee for Quality Assurance should establish mechanisms that ensure that research on effective demonstrations informs more permanent health care reforms, including the development of accountability measures and payment models.

Recommendation 5e. To enable comparative research and evaluation, researchers, evaluators, and agencies that develop measures and standards (e.g., the National Quality Forum, the National Committee for Quality Assurance, and the Centers for Medicare & Medicaid Services) should develop a consensus on and use a common core of measures reflecting social risk and protective factors as well as key health and social outcome measures. These measures should not be limited to clinical or economic metrics, but should include patient-reported outcomes and other outcomes relevant to a range of stakeholders, including patients, families, caregivers, communities, social care organizations, health care organizations, and payers. The Agency for Healthcare Research and Quality should curate these measures in a publicly available item bank.

1

Introduction

In a well-known public health parable—the upstream–downstream story, credited to medical sociologist Irving Zola—the story's protagonist is standing alongside a river that is slowly filling with drowning people. The protagonist starts pulling each drowning person from the water, but finds the pace of saving drowning people an impossible one to keep. More importantly, the immediacy of the need also prevents the protagonist from traveling upstream to determine how these people have come to be in the river at all (McKinlay, 1979). This parable represents a fundamental challenge facing the U.S. health care delivery system, which largely focuses on downstream activities. The health care delivery system is primarily focused on providing medical interventions to treat or prevent disease, but is not currently equipped to systematically address the many upstream factors that contribute to illness and poor health care outcomes.[1]

While the upstream-downstream story is often interpreted as enjoining clinicians to focus on disease prevention as well as treatment of acute or chronic illness (e.g., focusing on the role of diet, physical activity, and tobacco use in the onset of heart disease, rather than only focusing on the treatment of heart disease that may occur as a consequence of these behaviors), more contemporary interpretations have suggested the need to move even further upstream. Taking the social conditions in which an individual lives, works, and plays into account is critical to improving both primary prevention and the treatment of acute and chronic illness

[1] For a detailed look at supporting data, see Bradley and Taylor (2013).

because social contexts influence the delivery and outcomes of health care as well as individual health-related behaviors (Bravemen et al., 2011; Williams et al., 2008).

A large and growing body of evidence suggests that these upstream social resources—such as access to stable housing, nutritious food, and reliable transportation—contribute to health outcomes (Dzau et al., 2017a; Health Research & Educational Trust, 2017; Kaiser and Cafer, 2018; Williams et al., 2008). For example, people of lower socioeconomic status (SES) have a higher burden of poor health than those of higher SES (Adler and Rehkopf, 2008; Bor et al., 2017), including both a higher prevalence of most diseases and worse outcomes (Daly, 2014). Such health inequities are unnecessary, avoidable, and unjust and are not explained by differences in access to medical services or by individuals' genetic and behavioral factors (Heiman, 2015; NASEM, 2019b). Improving social conditions is likely to reduce health disparities and improve the health of the overall U.S. population (Abbott and Elliott, 2017; CDC, 2018).

Changes both at the societal level (possibly requiring changes in national law and policies) and at the patient level (requiring the provision of social care) are necessary to improve social conditions. As an example, though many other industrialized nations spend less per capita on medical services that the United States does, they spend a larger proportion on social services relative to medical services, and their residents have better health and lead longer lives (Bradley et al., 2017; NRC and IOM, 2013; Papanicolas et al., 2018; Squires and Anderson, 2015) (see Figure 1-1).

This report explores how a range of health care sector activities can be focused on improving social conditions as components of a comprehensive strategy to improve the nation's health and well-being. The United States is not alone in examining how to provide care for the whole needs of its population. For example, the United Kingdom's National Health System is moving forward with integrating its health and social care systems (NHS, n.d.).

The charge to the study committee is presented below, followed by a description of the committee's approach to its charge. Next, background information is given on how social, economic, and environmental factors influence health. Last, a roadmap to the rest of the report is provided.

CHARGE TO THE COMMITTEE

A broad coalition of foundations, social work associations and educational institutions, and other organizations came together to develop the Statement of Task that the committee was charged with addressing. The committee's task was to examine the potential for integrating services addressing social needs and the social determinants of health (SDOH)

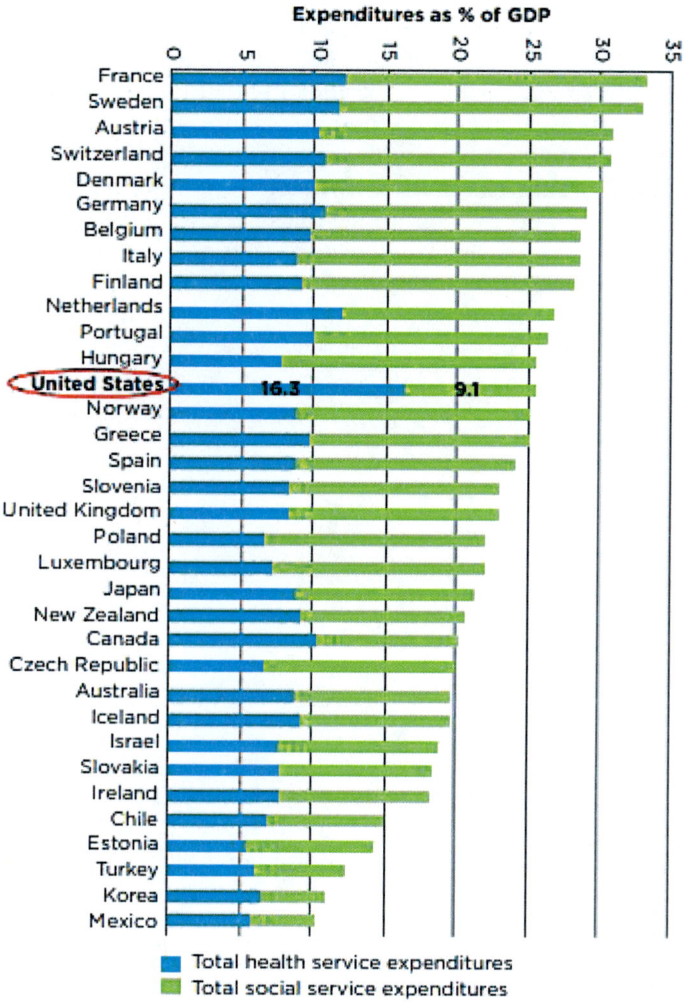

FIGURE 1-1 Health care and social services spending (percent of gross domestic product [GDP] across Organisation for Economic Co-operation and Development (OECD) countries.
SOURCE: Adapted from The American Health Care Paradox: Why Spending More Is Getting Us Less by Elizabeth H. Bradley, Lauren A. Taylor, and Harvey V. Fineberg, copyright © 2013, 2015. Reprinted by permission of PublicAffairs, an imprint of Hachette Book Group, Inc.

into the delivery of health care in order to achieve better health outcomes and to address major challenges facing the U.S. health care system. These challenges include persistent disparities in health outcomes between the overall population and certain vulnerable subpopulations, often defined by age, race, ethnicity, sex, gender identity, disability status, sexual orientation, SES, family caregiver status, immigrant status, or geographic location. In this report the committee discusses: (1) approaches currently being taken by health care providers and systems and also new or emerging approaches and opportunities; (2) the current roles of different disciplines and organizations as well as new or emerging roles and types of providers; and (3) current and emerging efforts to inform the design of an effective and efficient care system that will improve the nation's health and reduce health inequities. In creating its report, the committee considered the

1. Current scope and conceptual underpinnings of health-related social needs care,[2] including (a) the roles of providers such as social workers, gerontologists, physicians, psychologists, nurses, community health workers, and trained volunteers; (b) linkage to community-based organizations and services; and (c) the role of hospital community benefits.
2. Current state of the social needs care workforce in preventing, controlling, and treating health-related conditions (e.g., disciplines providing social needs care and their professional qualifications, the breadth of settings, and roles for such care, including administrative, policy, and research roles; current training for each discipline related to the provision of social needs care; and projected workforce needs to meet demographic changes).
3. Evidence of impact of social needs care on patient and caregiver/family health and well-being, patient activation, health care use, cost savings, and patient and provider satisfaction.
4. Opportunities and barriers to expanding historical roles and leadership of social workers in providing health-related social needs care and the expanding role of other types of providers, such as gerontologists.
5. Emerging and evidence-based care models that incorporate social workers or other social needs care providers in interprofessional care teams across the care continuum (e.g., acute, ambulatory, community-based, long-term care, hospice care, public health, care planning) and in delivery system reform efforts (e.g., enhancing

[2] The formal Statement of Task, included here, refers to "social needs care;" however, as noted in Table 1-2, the committee decided to use "social care."

prevention and functional status, care management, and transitional care; improving end-of-life care; integration of behavioral, mental, and physical health services).
6. Initiatives to improve population health and reform health care financing that incorporate social needs care (i.e., payments tied to quality metrics and alternative payment models, such as accountable care organizations, bundled payments, managed long-term services and supports, and accountable health communities).
7. Realized and potential contributions of social needs care to make health care delivery systems more community based, patient- and family/caregiver-centered, and responsive to social and structural determinants of health, particularly for vulnerable populations and communities, such as older adults and low-income families.
8. Opportunities for advancing the integration of social needs care services within community and health care delivery settings, such as expanding and improving interprofessional education; educating health care providers, payers, and patients about the benefits of social needs care services; and ensuring adequate reimbursement for said education by public and private payers.
9. Kinds of transdisciplinary research needed to understand the complex interplay of psychosocial and environmental factors on health, and to best inform efforts to develop policies and practices that lead to improved health outcomes.

The committee makes recommendations on how to (1) expand social needs care services; (2) better coordinate roles for social needs care providers in interprofessional care teams across the range of clinical and community health settings; and (3) optimize the effectiveness of social services to improve health and health care. Recommendations address areas such as the integration of services, training and oversight, workforce recruitment and retention, quality improvement, research and dissemination, and governmental and institutional policy for health care delivery and financing.

THE COMMITTEE'S APPROACH TO ITS CHARGE

The National Academies of Sciences, Engineering, and Medicine (the National Academies) appointed a committee of 18 subject-matter experts to carry out this task. The committee members have expertise in social work, nursing, gerontology, public health, clinical medicine, health law and policy, health services research, health care workforce, health care financing, and health insurance design.[3] The committee held four in-person meetings and two Web meetings over the course of the 18-month study to gather evidence, review and deliberate on the evidence, and develop conclusions and recommendations. To address this broad task, it was necessary to take into consideration several types of evidence, including peer-reviewed literature, reports from governmental agencies and private organizations (such as The Commonwealth Fund, the Institute for Healthcare Improvement, the Milbank Memorial Fund, the National Academies, the National Academy of Medicine, and the Robert Wood Johnson Foundation, among others), books, websites, and invited presentations to the committee during public sessions. Although the committee cast a wide net to identify relevant sources of information, it did not conduct a systematic literature review.

The purpose of the evidence review was to gain an understanding of opportunities for and barriers to integrating social care and health care and to identify both evidence-based and emerging approaches to such integration. Several literature searches were conducted. First, a broad search was conducted using key words related to the overarching topic areas of social work, social services, social welfare, the SDOH, care settings, models of care, integrated care, financing of care, workforce, quality assessment, and vulnerable populations, which were linked in various combinations using Boolean operators. Databases searched included Embase, Medline, Scopus, and Web of Science. The types of literature included peer-reviewed articles, reviews, grey literature reports, and conference proceedings. The websites of organizations conducting work in the area of social care were searched for relevant reports and papers. During the study, several narrowly defined literature searches were conducted to identify additional articles. Further information was gathered by querying committee members, representatives from the study sponsors, and others who work in the field. Studies of integration of health care and social care from nations other than the United States were not included in the review because of fundamental differences in how health care is delivered among nations and the inability to extrapolate findings from other countries to the United States. The committee aimed to identify the best available evidence, ideally evidence that included outcome data. Because integration of health care and social care is an area of active investigation and because assessment of emerging approaches is called out in the study charge, a variety of types of evidence, as noted above, were used as the evidence base to support findings and recommendations presented later in this report.

---

[3] Biographical information on the committee members can be found on the National Academies' website: https://www8.nationalacademies.org/pa/projectview.aspx?key=49935 (accessed May 15, 2019).

In conducting the study, the committee held three public sessions to obtain information and perspectives not readily available in the literature. The first public session was held on July 16, 2018, in Washington, DC, and provided an opportunity for the study sponsors and the committee members to discuss the Statement of Task, how the study supports the sponsoring organizations' missions, and, more broadly, why the study is important to carry out at this time. The second public session was held on September 24, 2018, in Washington, DC. The committee invited representatives from eight organizations to give presentations. Topics included the experiences of providing social care by several social service and health care organizations, support programs for family caregivers, and select federal government programs in support of providing social care. The third public session was held on November 13, 2018, via Web conference. During this public session, presentations focused on several social work–based models of care.

In addition to the public sessions noted above, the committee met five times in closed session to deliberate on the evidence and to develop findings and recommendations. Chapters 2–6 of this report summarize the evidence and present the committee's findings. Chapter 7 contains the committee's recommendations.

BACKGROUND

Inherent in the phrase "social determinants of health" is the implication that health is shaped by more than medical care. Defined by the World Health Organization (WHO) as "the conditions in which people are born, grow, live, work and age" (WHO, 2010), the SDOH have been conceptualized in terms of a socioecological model in which the person is at the center of micro, meso, and macro spheres of external influence (Dahlgren and Whitehead, 1991) (see Figure 1-2).[4] These radiating spheres reflect the second part of WHO's definition of the SDOH as being "shaped by the distribution of money, power, and resources at global, national, and local levels" (WHO, 2010).

Importantly, the SDOH are often misinterpreted as being negative or meant to apply only to a select group of people. All people experience social factors that influence their health. Some of these factors contribute favorably to health outcomes and others negatively. *Healthy People 2020* categorizes these interrelated determinants in five groups (see Table 1-1).[5]

---

[4] For more information related to the social determinants of health and conceptual socioecologic models, see Andersen, 1995; Bradley and Corwyn, 2002; and Taormina and Gao, 2013.

[5] Chapter 2 includes a discussion on screening for social determinants of health and the Appendix contains a list of screening tools for social determinants of health.

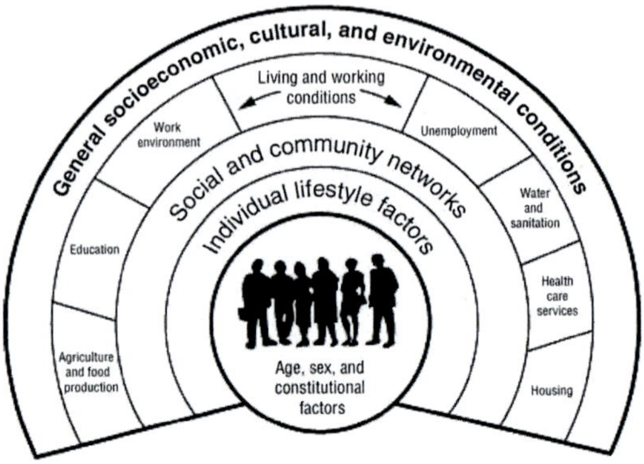

FIGURE 1-2 The Dahlgren-Whitehead model of social determinants of health.
SOURCE: Reprinted from Dahlgren G, Whitehead M. (1991). Policies and Strategies to Promote Social Equity in Health. Stockholm, Sweden: Institute for Futures Studies.

TABLE 1-1
Five Key Areas of Social Determinants of Health

Social Determinant of Health	Examples of Underlying Factors
Economic stability	Employment Food insecurity Housing instability Poverty
Education	Early childhood education and development Enrollment in higher education High school graduation Language and literacy
Social and community context	Civic participation Discrimination Incarceration Social cohesion
Health and health care	Access to health care Access to primary care Health literacy
Neighborhood and built environment	Access to foods that support healthy eating patterns Crime and violence Environmental conditions Quality of housing

SOURCE: HHS, 2019.

At their best, these SDOH can be protective of good health and wellness. For many people, however, the SDOH include a pattern of social risk factors that contribute to increased morbidity and mortality. The specific factors in each of the five categories that influence health in one way or another—and the ways in which the various factors interact—have been reviewed in multiple prior publications. Together these have contributed to an in-depth understanding of what causes and perpetuates vulnerability as well as of how these risks vary across the life course (e.g., see AARP Foundation, 2012; Acton and Malathum, 2000; Adler and Rehkopf, 2008; Bastos and Machado, 2013; Berkman et al., 2011; Blazer et al., 2007; Bor et al., 2017; Center for Surveillance, 2017; Collins et al., 1998; Council for Disabled Children, 2016; Diez Roux et al., 2001; Dzau et al., 2017b; Eriksson, 2011; Greenstone et al., 2013; Hummer and Hernandez, 2013; Kindig and Stoddart, 2003; Long et al., 2017; NASEM, 2019a,b; National Center for Injury Prevention and Control, 2018; NCEH, 2015; Sachs-Ericsson et al., 2006; Silverman, 2009; South et al., 2018; Thompson et al., 2019; Tobin-Tyler and Teitelbaum, 2018; VCU Center on Society and Health, 2014; Williams, 2013; Williams and Collins, 2001).

The consistent and compelling evidence on how social determinants shape health has led to a growing recognition throughout the health care sector that improving health and reducing health disparities is likely to depend—at least in part—on improving social conditions and decreasing social vulnerability. The gradual shift in the health care sector toward value-based payment incentivizes prevention and improved health and health care outcomes for persons and populations rather than service delivery alone. The combined result of these changes has been a growth in opportunities for health care systems to utilize the social and community contexts of patients with the aim of improving health outcomes. Some of these opportunities depend on the capacity of health care systems to link individual patients with government and community social services. Others are more focused on community-level social conditions. But important questions need to be answered about when and how health care systems should be involved in both providing social care and, more broadly, influencing social conditions—and what kinds of infrastructure and technical assistance would be required to facilitate these activities. At both the individual patient level and community level, this work is likely to require more deliberate alignment across sectors through such things as formal business arrangements, data sharing, payment policy and financial arrangements, and, where necessary, enabling legislation and regulation. Table 1-2 defines important terms used throughout the report.

TABLE 1-2
Key Terms Used in This Report

Health	A state of complete physical, mental, and social well-being and not merely the absence of disease or infirmity; this includes affording everyone the fair and just opportunity to be as healthy as possible.
Social care	Activities that address health-related social risk factors and social needs.
Social determinants of health	The conditions in which people are born, grow, work, live, and age that affect a wide range of health, functional, and quality of life outcomes and risks.
Social needs	A patient-centered concept that incorporates a person's perception of his or her own health-related needs.
Social risk factors	Social determinants that may be associated with negative health outcomes, such as poor housing or unstable social relationships.
Social services	Services, such as housing, food, and education, provided by government and private, profit and non-profit, organizations for the benefit of the community and to promote social well-being.

SOURCES: Adapted from Alderwick and Gottlieb, 2019; HHS, 2019; WHO, 2010.

ORGANIZATION OF THE REPORT

To respond to its charge, the committee examined ways in which health care delivery systems have increased activities to understand and intervene in social conditions as a strategy for improving health. It also examined the structural barriers to these activities. The committee's report is organized into six chapters beyond this one. Chapter 2 describes five complementary activities—awareness, adjustment, assistance, alignment, and advocacy—that health care systems can adopt to strengthen social care integration. Chapters 3–5 cover three system-level elements necessary to implement and sustain social care. Specifically, Chapter 3 describes the elements of a workforce that has the capability and capacity to improve social care within the five activities and the importance of using a collaborative approach. Chapter 4 describes how data and digital tools can be used to integrate social care and health care. Chapter 5 describes options for financing social care within the scope of health care. Chapter 6 describes challenges to implementing awareness, adjustment, and assistance strategies in health care delivery settings. Chapter 7 presents the committee's recommendations. The Appendix is a summary table of tools used for social needs screening.

REFERENCES

AARP Foundation, K. Elder, and J. Retrum. 2012. *Framework for isolation in adults over 50*. https://www.aarp.org/content/dam/aarp/aarp_foundation/2012_PDFs/AARP-Foundation-Isolation-Framework-Report.pdf (accessed May 24, 2019).

Abbott, L. S., and L. T. Elliott. 2017. Eliminating health disparities through action on the social determinants of health: A systematic review of home visiting in the United States, 2005–2015. *Public Health Nursing* 34(1):2–30.

Acton, G. J., and P. Malathum. 2000. Basic need status and health-promoting self-care behavior in adults. *Western Journal of Nursing Research* 22(7):796–811.

Adler, N. E., and D. H. Rehkopf. 2008. U.S. disparities in health: Descriptions, causes, and mechanisms. *Annual Review of Public Health* 29:235–252.

Alderwick, H., and L. M. Gottlieb. 2019. Meanings and misunderstandings: A social determinants of health lexicon for health care systems. *The Milbank Quarterly* 97(2):407–419.

Andersen, R. M. 1995. Revisiting the behavioral model and access to medical care: Does it matter? *Journal of Health and Social Behavior* 36(1):1–10.

Bastos, A., and C. Machado. 2009. Child poverty: A multidimensional measurement. *International Journal of Social Economics* 36(3):237–251.

Berkman, N. D., S. L. Sheridan, K. E. Donague, D. J. Halpern, and K. Crotty. 2011. Low health literacy and health outcomes: An updated systematic review. *Annals of Internal Medicine* 155(2):97–107.

Blazer, D. G., N. Sachs-Ericsson, and C. F. Hybels. 2007. Perception of unmet basic needs as a predictor of depressive symptoms among community-dwelling older adults. *Journal of Gerontology* 62A(2):191–195.

Bor, J., G. H. Cohen, and S. Galear. 2017. Population health in an era of rising income inequality: USA, 1980–2015. *The Lancet* 389(10077):1475–1490.

Bradley, E. H., H. Sipsma, and L. A. Taylor. 2017. American health care paradox: High spending on health care and poor health. *QJM: An International Journal of Medicine* 110(2):61–65.

Bradley, R. H., and R. F. Corwyn. 2002. Socioeconomic status and child development. *Annual Review of Psychology* 53:371–399.

Braveman, P., S. Egerter, and D. R. Williams. 2011. The social determinants of health: Coming of age. *Annual Review of Public Health* 32:381–398.

CDC (Centers for Disease Control and Prevention). 2018. *Social determinants of health: Know what affects health*. https://www.cdc.gov/socialdeterminants/index.htm (accessed May 24, 2019).

Center for Surveillance, Epidemiology, and Laboratory Services. 2017. *About rural health*. Centers for Disease Control and Prevention. https://www.cdc.gov/ruralhealth/about.html (accessed May 24, 2019).

Collins, J. W., Jr., R. J. David, R. Symons, A. Handler, S. Wall, and S. Andes. 1998. African-American mothers' perception of their residential environment, stressful life events, and very low birthweight. *Epidemiology* 9(3):286–289.

Council for Disabled Children. 2016. *Identifying the social care needs of disabled children and young people and those with SEN as part of education, health, and care needs assessments*. https://councilfordisabledchildren.org.uk/sites/default/files/field/attachemnt/Identifying%20the%20social%20care%20needs_0.pdf (accessed May 24, 2019).

Dahlgren, G., and M. Whitehead. 1991. *Policies and strategies to promote social equity in health*. Institute for Futures Studies. https://core.ac.uk/download/pdf/6472456.pdf (accessed May 26, 2019).

Daly, M. 2014. A social rank explanation of how money influences health. *Health Psychology* 34(3):222–230.

Diez Roux, A. V., S. S. Merkin, D. Arnett, L. Chambless, M. Massing, F. J. Nieto, P. Sorlie, M. Szklo, H. A. Tyroler, and R. L. Watson. 2001. Neighborhood of residence and incidence of coronary heart disease. *New England Journal of Medicine* 345(2):99–106.

Dzau, V. J., M. B. McClellan, J. M. McGinnis, S. P. Burke, M. J. Coye, A. Diaz, T. A. Daschle, W. H. Frist, M. Gaines, M. A. Hamburg, J. E. Henney, S. Kumanyika, M. O. Leavitt, R. M. Parker, L. G. Sandy, L. D. Schaeffer, G. D. Steele, Jr., P. Thompson, and E. Zerhouni. 2017a. Vital directions for health and health care: Priorities from a National Academy of Medicine initiative. *JAMA* 317(14):1461–1470.

Dzau, V. J., M. McClellan, J. M. McGinnis, and E. M. Finkelman (eds.). 2017b. *Vital directions for health & health care: An initiative of the National Academy of Medicine*. Washington, DC: National Academy of Medicine.

Eriksson, M. 2011. Social capital and health: Implications for health promotion. *Global Health Action* 4:5611.

Greenstone, M., A. Looney, J. Patashnick, and M. Yu. 2013. *Thirteen economic facts about social mobility and the role of education*. The Hamiliton Project, The Brookings Institution. https://www.brookings.edu/wp-content/uploads/2016/06/THP_13EconFacts_FINAL.pdf (accessed May 26, 2019).

Health Research & Educational Trust. 2017. *Housing and the role of hospitals*. Social Determinants of Health Series, American Hospital Association. https://www.aha.org/ahahret-guides/2017-08-22-social-determinants-health-series-housing-and-role-hospitals (accessed July 12, 2019).

Heiman, H. 2015. *Beyond health care: Role of social determinants in promoting health and health equity*. Kaiser Family Foundation. http://files.kff.org/attachment/issue-brief-beyond-health-care (accessed May 26, 2019).

HHS (U.S. Department of Health and Human Services). 2019. *Healthy people 2020: Social determinants of health*. https://www.healthypeople.gov/2020/topics-objectives/topic/social-determinants-of-health (accessed May 8, 2019).

Hummer, R. A., and E. M. Hernandez. 2013. The effect of educational attainment on adult mortality in the United States. *Population Bulletin* 68(1):1–16.

Kaiser, M. L., and A. Cafer, 2018. Understanding high incidence of severe obesity and very low food security in food pantry clients: Implications for social work. *Social Work in Public Health* 33(2):125–139.

Kindig, D., and G. Stoddart. 2003. What is population health? *American Journal of Public Health* 93(3):380–383.

Long, P., M. Abrams, A. Milstein, G. Anderson, K. Lewis Apton, M. Lund Dahlberg, and D. Whicher (eds.). 2017. *Effective care for high-need patients: Opportunities for improving outcomes, value, and health*. Washington, DC: National Academy of Medicine.

McKinlay, J. 1979. A case of refocusing upstream: The political economy of illness. In E. G. Jaco (ed.), *Patients, physicians, and illness. A sourcebook in behavioral science and health, 3rd ed*. London, UK: The Free Press. Pp. 9–25.

NASEM (National Academies of Sciences, Engineering, and Medicine). 2019a. *The promise of adolescense: Realizing opportunity for all youth*. Washington, DC: The National Academies Press.

NASEM. 2019b. *Vibrant and healthy kids: Aligning science, practice, and policy to advance health equity*. Washington, DC: The National Academies Press.

National Center for Injury Prevention and Control. 2018. *The social-ecological model: A framework for prevention*. Centers for Disease Control and Prevention. https://www.cdc.gov/violenceprevention/overview/social-ecologicalmodel.html (accessed August 12, 2018).

NCEH (National Center for Environmental Health). 2015. *CDC's built environment and health initiative*. https://www.cdc.gov/nceh/information/built_environment.htm. Last Modified: December 8, 2015 (accessed May 24, 2019).

NHS (National Health Service) England. n.d. *Integrated care systems.* https://www.england.nhs.uk/integratedcare/integrated-care-systems (accessed July 12, 2019).

NRC and IOM (National Research Council and Institute of Medicine). 2013. *U.S. health in international perspective: Shorter lives, poorer health.* Washington, DC: The National Academies Press.

Papanicolas, I., L. R. Woskie, and A. K. Jha. 2018. Health care spending in the United States and other high-income countries. *JAMA* 319(10):1024–1039.

Sachs-Ericsson, N., C. Schatschneider, and D. G. Blazer. 2006. Perception of unmet basic needs as a predictor of physical functioning among community-dwelling older adults. *Journal of Aging and Health* 18(6):852–868.

Silverman, M. 2009. Issues in access to healthcare by transgender individuals. *Women's Rights Law Reporter* 30(2):347–351.

South, E. C., B. C. Hohl, M. C. Kondo, J. M. MacDonald, and C. C. Branas. 2018. Effect of greening vacant land on mental health of community-dwelling adults: A cluster randomized trial. *JAMA Network Open* 1(3):e180298.

Squires, D., and C. Anderson. 2015. U.S. health care from a global perspective: Spending, use of services, prices, and health in 13 countries. *Issue Brief (Commonwealth Fund)* 15:1–15.

Taormina, R. J., and J. H. Gao. 2013. Maslow and the motivation hierarchy: Measuring satisfaction of the needs. *American Journal of Psychology* 126(2):155–177.

Thompson, T., A. McQueen, M. Croston, A. Luke, N. Caito, K. Quinn, J. Funaro, and M. W. Kreuter. 2019. Social needs and health-related outcomes among Medicaid beneficiaries. *Health Education and Behavior* 46(3):436–444.

Tobin-Tyler, E., and J. Teitelbaum. 2018. *Essentials of health justice: A primer*. Burlington, MA: Jones & Bartlett Learning.

VCU (Virginia Commonwealth University) Center on Society and Health. 2014. *Why education matters to health: Exploring the causes.* https://societyhealth.vcu.edu/media/society-health/pdf/test-folder/CSH-EHI-Issue-Brief-2.pdf (accessed May 26, 2019).

WHO (World Health Organization). 2010. *About social determinants of health.* https://www.who.int/social_determinants/sdh_definition/en (accessed May 24, 2019).

Williams, D. R., and C. Collins. 2001. Racial residential segregation: A fundamental cause of racial disparities in health. *Public Health Reports* 116(5):404–416.

Williams, D. R., M. C. Costa, A. O. Odunlami, and S. A. Mohammed. 2008. Moving upstream: How interventions that address the social determinants of health can improve health and reduce disparities. *Journal of Public Health Management & Practice* 14:S8–S17.

Williams, J. 2013. Social care and older prisoners. *Journal of Social Work* 13(5):471–491.

2

Five Health Care Sector Activities to Better Integrate Social Care

Health care sector leaders often make decisions about improving social care through care integration and investment in the absence of information about different strategies (Alderwick et al., 2018; Bickerdike et al., 2017; De Milto and Nakashian, 2016; Gottlieb et al., 2017b; Institute for Alternative Futures, 2012). An evidence-informed taxonomy of health care–based strategies that can be used to support and strengthen integration may help guide activities in this area.

Based on the existing literature and other sources, as described in Chapter 1, the committee identified five mutually complementary categories of activities that health systems can adopt to strengthen integration (see Figure 2-1). While all of the categories will ultimately benefit patients, two of these (*adjustment* and *assistance*) focus on improving care delivery provided specifically to individual patients based on information about their social risks and protective factors (conditions or attributes that may mitigate or eliminate risk). Two others (*alignment* and *advocacy*) relate to roles that the health care sector can play in influencing and investing in social care resources at the community level. All of these delivery and community-level activities are informed by efforts that increase *awareness* (the fifth category) of individual or community-level socioeconomic risks and assets relevant to a health system's geographic region or served population. Health care stakeholders—including providers, care delivery organizations, health plans, and government payers—that are exploring opportunities to launch or strengthen integration should understand the challenges of and interplay among these different strategies as well as the range of activities possible within each category. Each of

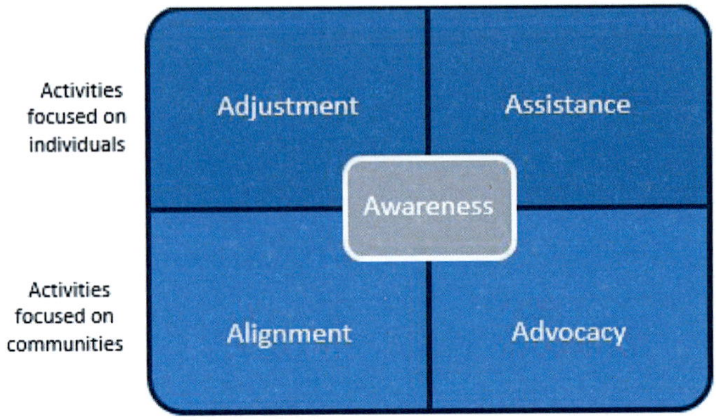

FIGURE 2-1 Health care system activities that strengthen social care integration.

the five categories (awareness, adjustment, assistance, alignment, and advocacy) depends on systems-level changes to implement and sustain integration—including a defined and well-trained workforce, data and digital tool innovations, and new financing models. These systems-level elements are the focus of subsequent chapters of this report.

HEALTH CARE ACTIVITIES TO STRENGTHEN SOCIAL CARE AND HEALTH CARE INTEGRATION

The five complementary types of integration activities correspond to different roles that health systems can play to strengthen the delivery of social care in health care settings. These activities build on the community-informed and patient-centered care[1] recommendations from a previous National Academies of Sciences, Engineering, and Medicine (the National Academies) report, *Systems Practices for the Care of Socially At-Risk Populations* (NASEM, 2016) (see Figure 2-2), by illustrating how these two approaches can most efficiently interact to enable high-quality care, whether to keep people healthy or reduce the burden of disease.

In developing its overall strategy to social care integration, the committee drew on this report's overarching theme—moving upstream to

---

[1] *Patient-centered care* is defined as providing care that is respectful of and responsive to individual patient preferences, needs, and values, and ensuring that patient values guide all clinical decisions (IOM, 2001).

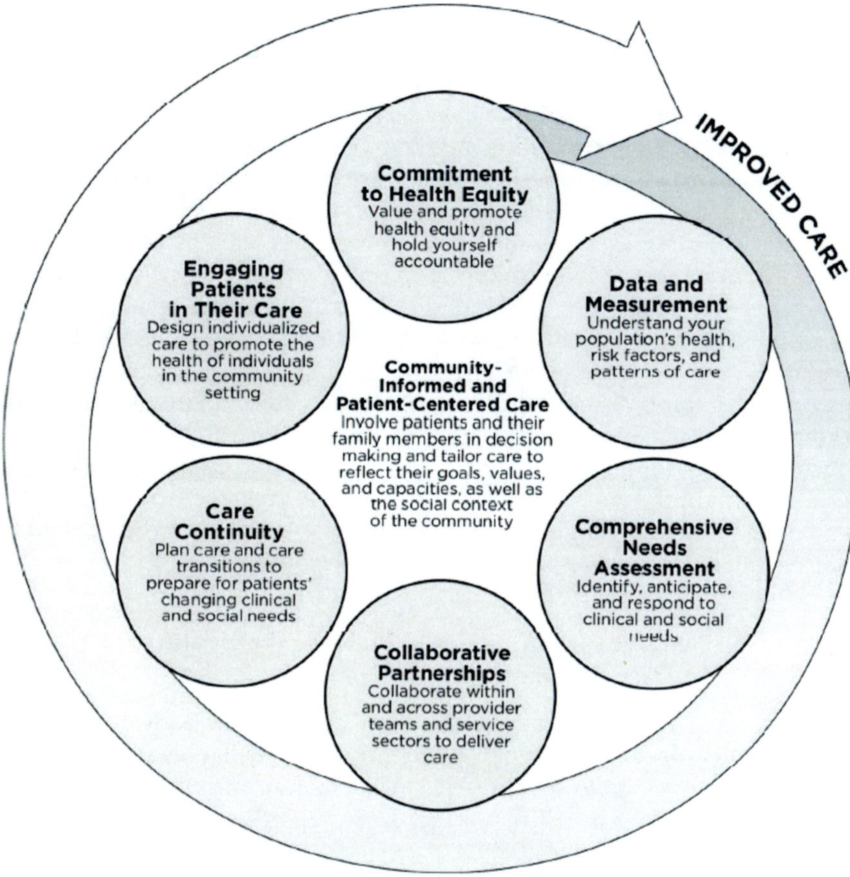

FIGURE 2-2 Promising systems practices to improve care for socially at-risk populations.
SOURCE: NASEM, 2016.

improve the nation's health—and recognized that there are both "near" and "far" upstream activities for strengthening integration. Near-upstream activities are targeted toward interactions that individuals have with health care clinical providers or clinical systems, whether for primary prevention or treatment of acute and chronic illness. They include ensuring that health care providers adjust traditional medical care decision making based on social risk and assets data and that patients with social risk factors then receive assistance connecting with and securing available government and community resources related to identified social needs. Far-upstream activities are more community-oriented. They involve aligning health care resources and investments to facilitate collaborations with community and government sectors as well as bringing health care assets into broader advocacy activities that augment and strengthen social care resources. As an example of how this could work in practice, Table 2-1 describes ways in which individuals' access to transportation might be improved using the five categories of activities.

The five broad categories are not part of a sequential process; they instead complement one another, and health care stakeholders might engage in multiple strategies simultaneously. These categories provide multiple pathways to achieving integration based on the evidence considered by the committee. Therefore, it would be a disservice to the field to suggest rules, guidelines, or a one-size-fits-all approach because one size does not fit all. Any of these categories is an umbrella for many specific activities that may take different forms, including similar activities that involve different levels of intensity. For example, assistance programs can range from light touch (e.g., providing patient handouts with basic information about social resources) to high touch (offering intensive case management to patients who need more help obtaining resources). These activities are described in more detail below, accompanied by relevant examples.

Awareness: Strategies to Increase the Health Care Sector's Awareness of Social Risks

Both national and local health sector activities seeking to increase social and health care integration frequently begin with elevating and sustaining awareness about the influence of social risk and protective factors

TABLE 2-1
Transportation-Related Examples Highlighting Different Categories of Social and Health Care Integration Activities

Awareness			
Ask people about their access to transportation.			
Adjustment	**Assistance**	**Alignment**	**Advocacy**
Reduce the need for in-person health care appointments by using other options such as telehealth appointments.	Provide transportation vouchers so that patients can travel to health care appointments. Vouchers can be used for ride-sharing services or public transit.	Invest in community ride-sharing or time-bank programs.	Work to promote policies that fundamentally change the transportation infrastructure within the community.

on health outcomes. Across both social and health sectors, the general awareness of the relevance of social factors on health is increasing rapidly. The committee documented an exponential increase in medical literature published over the past 18 years that (1) refers to the social determinants of health (SDOH); and (2) links those determinants with health care delivery (see Figure 2-3).

The committee defined *awareness* as those activities that identify the social risks and assets of defined patients and populations. Awareness strategies are not limited to sector-level awareness of the intersection of social risks and health outcomes. Instead, the committee recognized that building stakeholders' investments in social care also involves a more active, immediate awareness of a specific population's social risks and assets. Though the committee acknowledged that awareness is an important component of both individual- and community-level activities aimed at improving care integration, no consensus exists regarding the most effective or efficient strategies to increase awareness in ways that can facilitate subsequent actions. The strategies that health care systems already invest in to increase awareness vary across settings. The Kaiser Permanente Social Needs Network for Evaluation and Translation (SONNET) has highlighted five different pathways through which information about social risks and assets can be brought to the attention of health care systems (see

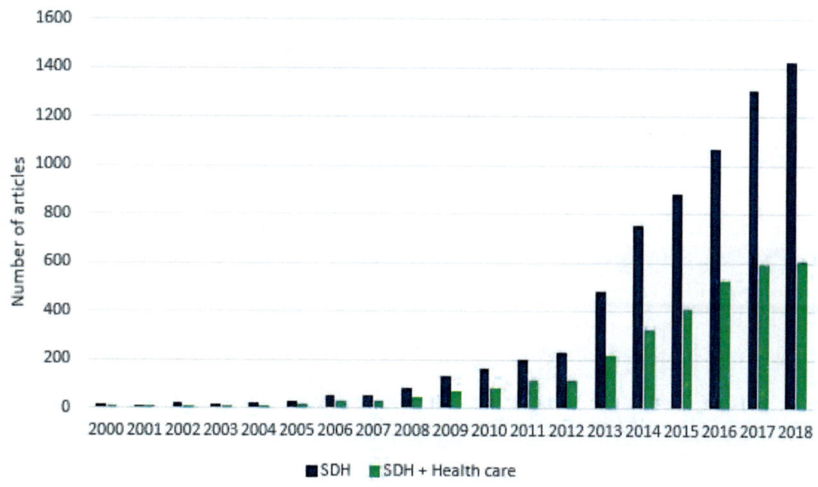

FIGURE 2-3 PubMed search results for "social determinants of health" overall and in the context of health care, 2000–2018.
NOTES: Number of results of PubMed searches for "social determinants of health" (SDH) and for "social determinants of health AND health care" (SDH + Health care). Search performed by the committee on January 15, 2019.
SOURCE: Adapted from Gottlieb et al., 2017a.

Figure 2-4): clinical care, screening large populations, screening high-risk groups, hotspotting, and identifying vulnerable communities.

On the clinical side, patients visiting health care organizations are increasingly being asked to answer social risk screening questions in the context of their care and care planning. In some places, screening is incentivized by payers. As part of the MassHealth Medicaid program, for instance, Massachusetts accountable care organizations now include social screening as a measure of care quality (MassHealth, 2018a,b). Similar initiatives are under way in North Carolina and Rhode Island. Clinic-based screening can be universal (everyone in a health care setting is asked about social risks, such as housing or food, either at each visit or at defined intervals; see Pathway 1 in Figure 2-4), or it can be more directed at specific age groups (e.g., children and seniors) or high-risk groups (e.g., people with certain diseases or who are on government insurance) (see Pathways 2 and 3 in Figure 2-4). As an example, Geisinger Health directs food security screening and interventions specifically at patients with diabetes (Feinberg et al., 2017). It is important to note that efforts to raise awareness by collecting data (both on patient clinical history and overall community health) may be affected by unconscious or implicit biases held by program leaders and practitioners, which can create new implementation barriers and workforce training demands (detailed further in Chapters 3 and 6) (Garg et al., 2005; Gottlieb and Alderwick, 2019).

A wide array of social risk screening tools has emerged to meet the demand for clinic-based social risk awareness activities (UCSF, 2019). Existing screening tools vary in the social domains covered, length, language accessibility, and other characteristics (UCSF, 2019) (see Table A-1 for adult screening tools; pediatric screening tools also are available).

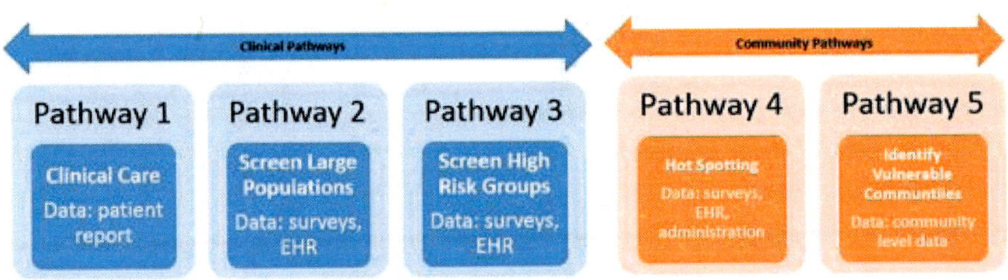

FIGURE 2-4 Pathways to identify basic resource needs.
NOTE: EHR = electronic health record
SOURCE: Steiner JF, Adams JL, Clausen D, Clift KM, Millan A, Nau CL, Roblin D, Schmittdiel JA, Schroeder EB. Predictive Models for Social Determinants of Health in KP Members and Communities: An Issue Brief from Kaiser Permanente's Social Needs Network for Evaluation and Translation (SONNET). Kaiser Permanente SONNET and Kaiser Permanente Community Health, September 2018.

Often these tools use different measures to assess social risks even under a single domain.

Though some screening tools use items from domain-specific validated instruments (e.g., hunger vital signs) (Hager et al., 2010), scant research is available on the psychometric validity of grouped items (Lewis et al., 2019). Existing studies generally indicate that a strong majority of patients find clinic-based social risk screening acceptable (Fleegler et al., 2007), though the unintended consequences (Garg et al., 2016) and possible opportunity costs of clinic-based screening have not been clearly articulated (NASDOH, 2019).

Some health systems use neighborhood- or community-level data to help select patients for more targeted social risk screening or to help identify high-risk communities (see Pathway 5 in Figure 2-4). For example, Cincinnati Children's Hospital conducts particularly intensive outreach with patients from two high-poverty zip codes to identify children with social needs (Auger et al., 2017). To facilitate such targeted outreach activities, the American Board of Family Medicine and the University of Missouri's Center for Applied Research and Engagement Systems have together developed the Population Health Assessment Engine (PHATE), which is provided to clinical providers enrolled in the American Board of Family Medicine's PRIME registry (American Board of Family Medicine, 2019). PHATE uses patient address data to incorporate "community vital signs" into patient charts based on publicly available census-tract-level characteristics. These and other uses of PHATE are summarized in Box 2-1. Some nonprofit hospitals, federally qualified health centers, and local public health departments also use the community-level social risk data in community health needs assessments, which are required by the Internal Revenue Service and are intended to influence community-level investments (Alberti et al., 2014).

The committee searched for indicators of the prevalence of awareness activities (e.g., social risk assessments or data linkages across social and medical sectors). Though multiple surveys targeting different health care stakeholders (e.g., payers, health systems executives, providers, and consumers) have asked about the prevalence of social screening in health care settings, there are limited data that can be synthesized across these surveys (findings from 23 surveys are summarized by SIREN) (Cartier et al., 2019). The majority of the existing surveys ask whether the health care system conducts some form of social risk assessment broadly without asking further questions about the specific strategies undertaken to obtain information. For example, survey items typically fail to distinguish among universal, clinic-based social screening, targeted screening for high-risk patients, and community data integration; they do not ask respondents to report the numbers of patients who complete social risk

Box 2-1 Uses of Population Health Assessment Engine

- Map physician or clinic service area
- Show clusters of disease
- Show clusters of poor outcomes
- Pull in social determinant data (poverty, less than high school education, single parent household, unemployment, etc.)
- Create a "community vital sign" for every patient
- Display community resources for patients and practice

The resulting reports and information help clinicians and practices better understand the characteristics of patient risks, illuminating local resources and opportunities for assistance, intervention, and improvement.

SOURCE: American Board of Family Medicine, 2019.

assessments; and they do not ask about the capacity of the workforce or activities undertaken in general or by discipline to respond to any identified risks. Some research has explored the adequacy of using electronic health record (EHR) documentation (e.g., LOINC, SNOMED, *International Statistical Classification of Diseases and Related Health Problems, 10th Revision* [ICD-10], Current Procedural Terminology [CPT] codes) to gauge the prevalence of individual-level social risk screening, though this would fail to capture other related activities that facilitate social needs and asset awareness. At this time, the lack of both coding standards and capacity in medical coding systems and documentation incentives makes EHRs an unreliable source of information (Arons et al., 2018; DeSilvey et al., 2018; Lewis et al., 2016; Navathe et al., 2018; Torres et al., 2017). These and other technology-based opportunities to strengthen care integration are the focus of Chapter 4.

In reviewing different strategies to increase the health care sector's awareness of patient and population social risk and protective factors, the committee went on to ask whether increasing the health care sector's recognition of social risks alone could contribute to changes in health outcomes in the absence of dedicated social care interventions. Specifically, does asking equate to an intervention? This question could be especially relevant to the awareness strategies in which individual patients are asked about their social risks in the context of a health care delivery encounter. Does asking about social risks without coupling screening activities with a related social care intervention, such as, at a minimum, making a referral for a patient to follow up at his or her discretion, affect the provider–patient relationship in some way? Could asking have negative consequences, such as triggering or creating trauma (Garg et al., 2016)? The committee did not find a strong body of evidence to support either positive or negative consequences of implementing awareness strategies in isolation. This is likely because there are few clinical systems implementing clinic-based screening without some form of intervention.

Even in settings when relevant interventions are offered, patients do not consistently desire assistance, making it important to consider shared decision-making principles as part of patient-centered care planning that results from identifying social risk factors and social needs (Swavely et al., 2018; Tong et al., 2018). Some research suggests that patients do not believe that social screening needs to be accompanied by interventions and may have salutary effects in isolation, although the evidence is mixed (Byhoff et al., in press; Palakshappa et al., 2017). As an example, patients' perceptions that they are receiving equity-oriented care—including care that is trauma-, culture-, and context-informed—are linked with comfort and confidence in care, which itself is associated with improved confidence in managing health problems (Ford-Gilboe et al., 2018). Lower rates of patient–provider discussions about social demographic circumstances were found to be associated with six times higher odds of poor medication adherence (Schoenthaler et al., 2017). More research is needed on how screening activities themselves affect patient–provider relationships.

Adjustment: Activities Where Social Risk Information Is Used to Inform Clinical Care Decision Making

There are many different ways in which an awareness of social risks (collected through any of the awareness strategies described above) can subsequently influence health care sector activities, leading to such things as providing social care coordination and services and augmenting the availability of social care resources (see assistance, alignment, and advocacy sections below). Social risk data also could be used to inform adjustments to care that focus not on resolving social risks directly but instead on altering clinical care to accommodate identified social barriers. Thus, social and economic barriers to high-quality care may be mitigated by changes to how the health care services are delivered in addition to any attempts to resolve the social risk itself.

Many examples of adjustment strategies were identified in the literature, including the delivery of language and literacy-concordant services; smaller doctor-patient panel sizes for cases with socially complex needs (e.g., teams caring for homeless patients in the U.S. Department of Veterans Affairs [VA] health system have panel sizes smaller than the size of other VA care teams); offering open-access scheduling or evening and weekend clinic access; and providing telehealth services, especially in rural areas (Felland et al., 2003; VA, 2019). Other examples of ways that providers can adjust care based on known social risks involve changing insulin dosages at the end of the month when food benefits are more likely to run out (Seligman et al., 2014) and shifting to indoor or supervised physical activity recommendations for patients who live in unsafe neighborhoods (Waite, 2018). These adjustments can have a significant impact; for instance, providing last-shift or overnight dialysis beds, offering longer acting anti-hypertensive medications, or changing visit schedules may improve outcomes in homeless patients with end-stage renal disease (Holley et al., 2006; Podymow and Turnbull, 2013). These examples highlight adaptations to traditional care designed to accommodate patients' social contexts but are not interventions focused on changing the underlying social risk.

The amount of evidence suggesting that adjustment interventions affect health varies depending on the type of intervention because there are many different activities in this general category. For example, a strong body of evidence supports providing interpreter services, which can be considered a form of adjusted care delivery since care modifications (as opposed to English classes) are provided based on an understanding of patient social and cultural characteristics that can be gained through better communication (Ku and Flores, 2005; Wasserman et al., 2014). As described in the awareness section above, some evidence suggests that context-informed care can influence patients' experience of care, health behaviors, and health outcomes. Health services researchers have described clinical care that incorporates an understanding of social context as "contextualized care" (Weiner et al., 2010). And while there is a relevant, intersecting body of evidence on shared decision making and patient-centered care approaches, research in those areas has not consistently and explicitly focused on care modifications or interventions that mitigate the impacts of social and economic adversity (Sambare et al., 2017).

Social risk–adjusted payments also could be considered adjustment strategies if they are not linked explicitly to requirements like social care coordination or housing supports. Massachusetts is currently experimenting with Medicaid capitation rates that change based on patients' social risks (e.g., neighborhood deprivation and housing status) (Breslin et al., 2017; Commonwealth of Massachusetts, 2017; Crumley and Marlise, 2018). Chapter 5 provides more details about risk-adjusted payments.

The increased focus on the intersection of social risk and health outcomes at a national level provides an opportunity to recognize, evaluate, and potentially incentivize contextualized care so that it can be implemented more systematically throughout the U.S. health care sector. The adjustment approach to social care integration is potentially the least controversial of health care strategies to strengthen social care since the focus of care remains within the traditional wheelhouse of medical care. Nonetheless, substantial gaps in knowledge exist about how adjustment strategies should affect disease-specific care decisions. For example, though many expert care guidelines on diabetes, hypertension, and obesity recognize the influence of social context, sparse information is provided in those social guidelines about how providers should alter their care based on specific social risks (American Diabetes Association, 2017; Armstrong and Joint National Committee, 2014; Eckel et al., 2014; Jensen et al., 2014; Stone et al., 2014). Thus, it is not surprising that some research shows that clinical care is not systematically context-informed in U.S. health care settings. When social risk data are provided via verbal cues, for instance, providers inconsistently incorporate the information into care decisions (Levinson et al., 2000; Tong et al., 2018; Weiner et al., 2010). In one study, providers given verbal cues about patients' complex contextual circumstances subsequently provided contextually appropriate care in less than 23 percent of cases (Weiner et al., 2010). Health care workers may resist universal screening given the limited evidence on how to screen most effectively, insufficient support for referrals and follow up, and changes in procedures and workflow that may be necessitated by screening.

There are many outstanding questions about whether there should be more explicit adjustments to care recommended for patients with specific social risks (e.g., food or housing insecurity) in order to maximize the uptake of guideline-concordant care. For instance, the potential for such adjustments to widen rather than lessen health inequities must be considered. Concerns have arisen from concrete examples in the health care system where social risk factors have been wielded to deny evidence-based care to select populations. For instance, history suggests African Americans have been systematically denied adequate pain management due to both conscious and unconscious biases about pain perception and racialized depictions of addiction, substance abuse, social support, and a perceived inability to comply with pain management practices (Primm et al., 2004). To avoid such discrimination caused by the presence of social risks, new care management guidelines must be thoughtfully designed both to incorporate social risks into personalized care and to provide guardrails against discrimination. As these guidelines emerge, appropriately applying them will require relevant training curricula and incentives (Weiner and Schwartz, 2016). Training of the social care workforce is discussed in Chapter 3, and payment and financing reform that can support this work is the focus of Chapter 5.

Assistance: Strategies to Link Patients with Social Needs to Government and Community Resources

Beyond increasing awareness of patients' social risks and adjusting care to accommodate endorsed risks, there is a new focus on health care–based interventions on reducing social risk by providing assistance in connecting patients with relevant social care resources. The literature contains descriptions of a variety of assistance activities that have been undertaken by health systems and communities. These assistance activities vary in intensity, from lighter touch (one-time provision of resources, information, or referrals) to longer and more intensive interventions that attempt to assess and address patient-prioritized social needs more comprehensively (Bickerdike et al., 2017; Gottlieb et al., 2017b; Hannigan and Coffey, 2011).

Lighter-touch assistance activities can include providing information or vouchers for patients to obtain resources in the community (e.g., through curated resource lists) or referring patients to specific programs (e.g., to medical–legal partnerships to address legal barriers to housing or benefits, to eligibility counselors to enroll in Medicaid, or to social workers to obtain help with heating bills or short-term rental assistance). These lighter-touch interventions can include direct assistance (e.g., sending patients home with food if they report being hungry, providing rides directly to and from appointments, or offering respite care activities to support caregivers) (Berkowitz et al., 2018; Chaiyachati et al., 2018; Lindau et al., 2016; Martin et al., 2015).

More intensive assistance activities are often directed to medically and socially complex patients, and they typically include processes such as relationship building, comprehensive biopsychosocial needs assessments, care planning, interventions (e.g., resource connections, ongoing case management, and behavioral activation interventions, such as motivational interviewing), and long-term community-based supports (Burns and Essing, 2018; Lukens and McFarlane, 2004; Miller and Rollnick, 2012; NEJM Catalyst, 2017; Rizzo and Rowe, 2016). These more intensive assistance activities can enable the identification of co-occurring mental health concerns (such as low self-esteem, loneliness, and a history of trauma) and physical health barriers. As a result, intensive assistance activities can contribute to care adjustments at the same time as they are supporting the different processes. This has made the impacts of social care assistance activities difficult to disentangle from other intervention activities targeted at high-complexity patients (Gottlieb et al., 2017b). The AIMS care coordination model and the IMPaCT model are two examples of a higher-intensity assistance approach (see Box 2-2).

Assistance is sometimes provided directly by clinical care team members, such as primary care providers or registered nurses. Other times,

Box 2-2 Examples of High-Intensity Assistance Activities

AIMS: A Care Coordination Model

Goal: Address barriers to health and well-being by identifying medical and nonmedical risks and addressing priority needs in order to improve health, reduce the use of unnecessary health services, improve patient satisfaction with the health care delivery system, and help primary care providers maintain joy in work.

Approach: AIMS embeds master's-prepared social workers into primary and specialty care teams to assess the needs of complex patients and provide risk-focused care coordination. AIMS is implemented telephonically and/or in person and is typically completed in 6 to 8 weeks. Patients with nonmedical needs are identified by primary health care physicians or nurses and referred to the AIMS team members who deliver AIMS in four steps: patient engagement and assessment, care plan development, care management, and goal attainment. AIMS has also been replicated by community-based organizations in partnerships with local clinics.

Outcome: AIMS is integrated in seven primary care clinics at RUMC and has served several thousand patients since it was developed in 2010. AIMS patients were satisfied with health care services delivery and reported better ability to understand and manage their chronic illnesses. One retrospective evaluation revealed that AIMS patients had fewer hospital admissions, emergency department visits, and 30-day readmissions tchan patients in the broader RUMC population. A quasi-experimental study on AIMS found that recipients' health risks and depression scores were reduced within 6 months of the intervention, while the comparison group participants' scores were unchanged.

NOTE: AIMS = Ambulatory Integration of the Medical and Social; RUMC = Rush University Medical Center.
SOURCES: Rizzo et al., 2016; Rowe et al., 2019, in press.

IMPaCT Model (Individualized Management for Patient-Centered Targets)

Goal: Provide high-risk, low-income individuals with tailored social support, navigation of complex health systems, and advocacy to help them achieve their health goals.

Approach: Community health workers are hired from the local community to work with patients. The program is delivered in three stages: goal setting, short-term tailored supports, and connection with long-term supports.

Outcome: More than 6,000 people in Philadelphia, Pennsylvania, have been served by the program. In randomized trials, IMPaCT improved participants' access to primary care and mental health services; patient activation; and care quality. The program also reduced 30-day hospital readmissions. Outpatients with multiple chronic conditions that were enrolled in the program had improved chronic disease control and quality of care and reduced hospitalization.

SOURCE: Kangovi et al., 2018.

these activities are assigned to individuals whose roles are more focused on social care, such as social workers (Altfeld et al., 2012; Boutwell et al., 2016; Fabbre et al., 2011; Fraser et al., 2018; Gehlert et al., 2015; Rizzo and Rowe, 2016; Stanhope and Straussner, 2017), patient navigators, community health workers, or care coordinators (Berkowitz et al., 2018; Chinman et al., 2015; Dale et al., 2008; Gunderson et al., 2018; Kangovi et al., 2015; Repper and Carter, 2011; Salzer et al., 2010). These staff may be employed by health systems or by partner community-based organizations (Schrage, 2018). Systematically integrating assistance activities into health care organizations may necessitate changes in workflow, team dynamics, and organizational culture, and it may demand strategies to engage patients that depart from usual care. Together these requirements can present substantial barriers to implementation (Helfrich et al., 2016; also see Chapter 6).

Despite substantial evidence concerning the connection between social risks and health outcomes and use, there are few rigorously designed studies on the impact of assistance interventions on outcomes or use among participants (Gottlieb et al., 2017a). Rather, most evaluations of interventions have focused on process outcomes, such as patient satisfaction and self-reported health-related measures, and have not differentiated between specific intervention components (Gottlieb et al., 2017a). Moreover, many assistance interventions have evolved over time under principles of continuous quality improvement and learning health systems, using techniques such as pre–post analyses rather than more rigorous randomized control trials (McGinnis et al., 2014). Further research is needed in this area on the wide range of interventions that are and could be used to reduce patients' social risk. This research will need to more clearly articulate the added value of providing assistance services, particularly for specific populations who may report the same social need but have differing complexities and benefit eligibility that should inform assistance activities. The health care sector's approach of providing assistance with basic material needs, for instance, to patients who are medically complex is likely to differ from providing assistance to healthier populations.

Alignment and Advocacy: Activities Where Health Care Organizations Partner and Collaborate with Other Sectors

Increasingly, health care delivery organizations, health plans, and other health care stakeholders play roles in aligning health care assets with existing social care assets in communities and advocating for more social resources to improve community health and well-being. The committee defined alignment activities to include those undertaken by health care systems to understand existing social care assets in the community, organize them in such a way as to encourage synergy among the various activities, and invest in and deploy them to prevent emerging social needs and improve health outcomes. The committee defined advocacy activities as those in which health care organizations work with partner social care organizations to promote policies that facilitate the creation and redeployment of assets or resources in order to improve health outcomes and prevent emergence of unmet social needs. While providers, patients, and caregivers also can advocate to improve social resources for individual patients, the committee defined health care sector advocacy as activities that are aimed more broadly at increasing the availability of community resources for groups of patients. The net effect of both of these types of activities (alignment and advocacy) is to achieve what the Centers for Medicare & Medicaid Services defined as the objective of the alignment track of the Accountable Health Communities Model, which is to "optimize community capacity to address health-related social needs" (CMS, 2019).

In both the alignment and advocacy categories, health care organizations leverage their political, social, and economic capital within a community or local environment to encourage and enable health care and social care organizations to partner and pool resources, such as services and information, to achieve greater net benefit from the health care and social care services available in the community. Since 2009, reports from the Agency for Healthcare Research and Quality; the National Academies of Sciences, Engineering, and Medicine;[2] the U.S. Preventive Services Task Force; and other organizations have recommended improving the integration of clinical, public health, and community-based services and focusing on increasing the uptake of clinical preventive services (AHRQ, 2016; ASTHO, 2015; Dzau et al., 2017; IOM, 2012; Long et al., 2017; Ockene et al., 2007). Cross-sector collaboration is also a foundational strategy in the Robert Wood Johnson Foundation's Action Framework to build a Culture of Health and has been described in multiple reports on how partnership-driven work can integrate health care and social care services to improve population health (Plough, 2015; Towe et al., 2016). An important limitation of these collaborations is that they often occur in the context of uneven power dynamics and historical fragmentation between sectors due to differing funding sources and workforces.

Though such partnerships are not new, health care organizations are engaging in collaborative work in increasingly varied ways. However,

---

[2] As of March 2016, the Health and Medicine Division of the National Academies of Sciences, Engineering, and Medicine continues the consensus studies and convening activities previously carried out by the Institute of Medicine (IOM). The IOM name is used to refer to publications issued prior to July 2015.

despite national recommendations and increasing activity concerning the use of intersectoral work to strengthen community resources, the literature on the effectiveness of the health care sector's alignment and advocacy work in large part remains limited to case studies. Some evidence suggests that alignment and advocacy activities can improve a variety of health outcomes, from infection control to asthma and cardiovascular outcomes (Boex et al., 1998). One study demonstrating effectiveness found significantly lower death rates from potentially preventable conditions among communities with multi-sector networks supporting population health activities with alignment and advocacy strategies extending well beyond the boundaries of the traditional health care system to include policy changes supporting improved health outcomes (e.g., smoking bans and increasing access to healthy food) (Mays et al., 2016). Reporting bias may skew the literature toward positive outcomes narratives, including impacts on health care use, expenditures, and overall population-level health outcomes.

With the above caveats, a handful of illustrative examples are available to demonstrate three strategies that health care stakeholders have taken to increase alignment and advocacy in their communities.

1. *Partner with social care agencies to fill known gaps in services for beneficiaries.* One approach used by health care organizations to improve alignment and advocacy is to strengthen collaborations with social care organizations to directly provide needed services. For instance, the network Area Agencies on Aging coordinates with community-based organizations to provide community case management, home-delivered meals, and caregiver respite to aging populations (Brewster et al., 2018). This partnership formalized the referral infrastructure and established a compensation mechanism for these services that supports the assistance activities of the clinics while also aligning and investing in local resources and helping sustain and strengthen local, trusted institutions. In another example, the Henry Ford Health System partnered with Uber, Lyft, and Ford Motor Company to provide transportation to its patient population, with a particular focus on those in underserved communities (Knowles, 2018; Martinez, 2018). At the same time they are campaigning to modify existing transportation infrastructure in the city of Detroit in order to facilitate access in vulnerable communities. An increasing number of health care organizations are also investing in low-income housing. For example, UnitedHealth Group invested $50 million in low-income housing tax credit funds managed by the Greater Minnesota Housing Fund and Enterprise Community Investment,

resulting in the development of multi-family rental units for very low-income and special needs households (UnitedHealth Group, 2013).

2. *Develop anchor institution strategies.* A growing number of health care initiatives explore roles that the health care sector can play in improving the social, economic, and political landscape of local economies. In these cases, health care organizations adopt place-based, health-equity-focused strategies that recognize that social and economic determinants are largely responsible for health outcomes. These organizations often describe an "anchor mission" that helps them realign institutional assets to broadly combat social and economic disparities by investing in communities. Hospitals and health systems spend $782 billion annually, employ more than 5.6 million people, and hold investment portfolios of more than $400 billion (Ubhayakar et al., 2017). Investments made through anchor institution strategies sometimes rely on community development financial institutions, which provide access to capital often unavailable from traditional lenders, or on social impact bonds, in which case private funds are used to catalyze initiatives to address community needs. In 2019, more than 40 health care delivery organizations were participating in an anchor institution collaborative activity (Healthcare Anchor Network, 2019). For example, Rush University Medical Center's (RUMC's) anchor strategy involves hiring individuals from underserved communities to provide them with economic opportunity, establishing local and minority-owned business preferences for vendor and supply chain contracts, and creating a local financial investment strategy (Harkavy, 2016; Ubhayakar et al., 2017). As part of this approach, since 2017 RUMC has provided $6 million in loans to community development financial institutions, such as one supporting the city of Chicago's Neighborhood Rebuild Training pilot program. In programs like these the funding can be used in various aspects of the community, including renovations to homes in high crime areas and providing on-the-job training and credentialing opportunities to youth and ex-offenders (Chicago Community Loan Fund, 2018; Community Development Financial Institutions, 2019; RUMC, 2017). While it is difficult to gauge the impact of such long-term investments and collaborations, more outcome data will become available as more health care stakeholders undertake and report on their anchor activities. Another example is Stephen and Sandra Sheller 11th Street Family Health Services, a federally qualified health center in Philadelphia, Pennsylvania (Waite, 2018). 11th Street

works with neighborhood residents in cooperation with schools, churches, and community groups and agencies to provide for the biological, psychological, and social needs of its patients by offering a wide range of services, including creative arts therapies, fitness training, and nutrition classes.

3. *Organize and engage in cross-sector coalitions.* Other alignment and advocacy activity involves more actively organizing and engaging in multi-sector coalitions generally aimed at place-based community improvement. Johns Hopkins University, located in Baltimore, Maryland, is a member of the East Baltimore Development Initiative, a multi-stakeholder coalition seeking to revitalize the East Baltimore neighborhood (East Baltimore Development Inc., 2010). The university has engaged with the community through the Homewood Community Partners Initiative (HCPI) in 10 neighborhoods located around its main campus (JHU, 2019). HCPI has worked with the Central Baltimore Partnership, various community and neighborhood organizations, and other stakeholders, such as foundations and anchor institutions, to develop an implementation plan for the area. This plan contains 29 priority recommendations for action, including blight removal, housing and commercial development, and fundraising. From 2013 to 2016 Maryland established health enterprise zones in five communities to stimulate alignment and advocacy activities among local health departments, health care delivery organizations, and social care and community-based organizations; the effort resulted in a net cost savings of $93.39 million (across all zip codes that participated) due to reduced inpatient hospital visits (Gaskin et al., 2018). Hennepin Health, a Minnesota-based managed care program, reported similar notable gains coordinating assets at the county level, including across social care agencies, county-based health departments, multiple health systems, and a nonprofit health plan (Vickery et al., 2018). Together these agencies reported reductions in emergency department use and increased primary and preventative care use for Medicaid beneficiaries.

These strategies alone or in combination may be funded by health care organizations via community benefit programs—the required contributions that nonprofit health care delivery systems must make to earn their tax-exempt status.

The committee recognizes that health care organizations can bring funds, data, and political and other forms of capital to catalyze community activities—including through the various strategies described in this chapter. But the health care sector has not consistently wielded this capital in the interest of primary prevention of clinical conditions or prevention of the complicating social conditions. Effective strategies to strengthen social and health care integration are likely to require more attention to the experience and expertise of community stakeholders. This will demand organizational humility from the health care sector, particularly as it moves from health care delivery to community-focused activities. Alignment and advocacy initiatives should incorporate patients, families, and community members in program planning and execution to help avoid historical missteps.

As effective strategies emerge, attention will need to be given to implementation feasibility and program sustainability, including the workforce, technology, and payment models that will support the strategies and enable long-term interventions and corresponding reductions in health disparities.

FINDINGS

- Five complementary types of activities can facilitate the integration of social and health care. They are awareness, adjustment, assistance, alignment, and advocacy.
- These types of activities should not be considered mutually exclusive, and one does not necessarily build on another. The exception involves awareness activities, which typically are foundational to the others.
- Some health care systems have had success with using these strategies to strengthen social care services and, subsequently, to link social care activities with improved health outcomes.
- Robust outcome evaluations have not been conducted on social care integration activities, which limits the committee's ability to draw conclusions and make recommendations about specific evidence-based practices.
- A one-size-fits-all approach is neither feasible nor advisable, since context should influence the adoption of specific social and health care integration activities.

REFERENCES

AHRQ (Agency for Healthcare Research and Quality). 2016. *Clinical–community linkages.* https://www.ahrq.gov/professionals/prevention-chronic-care/improve/community/index.html (accessed February 7, 2019).

Alberti, P. M., K. Sutton, I. Baer, and J. Johnson. 2014. *Community health needs assessments: Engaging community partners to improve health.* Washington, DC: Association of American Medical Colleges.

Alderwick, H. A. J., L. M. Gottlieb, C. M. Fichtenberg, and N. E. Alder. 2018. Social prescribing in the U.S. and England: Emerging interventions to address patients' social needs. *American Journal of Preventive Medicine* 54(5):715–718.

Altfeld, S. J., E. Avery, R. L. Golden, T. J. Johnson, K. Karavolos, V. Nandi, M. Rooney, G. E. Shier, and A. J. Perry. 2012. Effects of an enhanced discharge planning intervention for hospitalized older adults: A randomized trial. *Gerontologist* 53(3):430–440.

American Board of Family Medicine. 2019. *PHATE: The Population Health Assessment Engine.* https://primeregistry.org/phate (accessed April 12, 2019).

American Diabetes Association. 2017. Standards of medical care in diabetes—2017, abridged for primary care providers. *Diabetes Care* 35(1):5–26.

Armstrong, C., and Joint National Committee. 2014. JNC8 guidelines for the management of hypertension in adults. *American Family Physician* 90(7):503–504.

Arons, A., S. DeSilvey, C. Fichtenberg, and L. Gottlieb. 2018. Documenting social determinants of health-related clinical activities using standardized medical vocabularies. *Journal of the American Medical Informatics Association Open.* doi: 10.1093/jamiaopen/ooy051.

ASTHO (Assocation of State and Territorial Health Officials). 2015. *Community–clinical linkages to improve hypertension identification, management, and control.* Issue brief. http://www.astho.org/Prevention/Community-Clinical-Linkages-Issue-Brief (accessed May 26, 2019).

Auger, K. A., R. S. Kahn, J. M. Simmons, B. Huang, A. N. Shah, K. Timmons, and A. F. Beck. 2017. Using address information to identify hardships reported by families of children hospitalized with asthma. *Academic Pediatrics* 17(1):79–87.

Berkowitz, S. A., S. Parashuram, K. Rowan, L. Andon, E. B. Bass, M. Bellantoni, D. J. Brotman, A. Deutschendorf, L. Dunbar, S. C. Durso, A. Everett, K. D. Giuriceo, L. Hebert, D. Hickman, D. E. Hough, E. E. Howell, X. Huang, D. Lepley, C. Leung, Y. Lu, C. G. Lyketsos, S. M. E. Murphy, T. Novak, L. Purnell, C. Sylvester, A. W. Wu, R. Zollinger, K. Koenig, R. Ahn, P. B. Rothman, P. M. C. Brown, and Johns Hopkins Community Health Partnership (J-CHiP) team. 2018. Association of a care coordination model with health care costs and utilization: The Johns Hopkins Community Health Partnership (J-CHiP). *JAMA Network Open* 1(7):e184273.

Bickerdike, L., A. Booth, P. M. Wilson, K. Farley, and K. Wright. 2017. Social prescribing: Less rhetoric and more reality. A systematic review of the evidence. *BMJ Open* 7(4):e013384.

Boex, J. R., J. Cooksey, and T. Inui. 1998. Hospital participation in community partnerships to improve health. *Joint Commission Journal on Quality Improvement* 24(10):541–548.

Boutwell, A. E., M. B. Johnson, and R. Watkins. 2016. Analysis of a social work–based model of transitional care to reduce hospital readmissions: Preliminary data. *Journal of the American Geriatrics Society* 64(5):1104–1107.

Breslin, E., A. Lambertino, D. Heaphy, and T. Dreyfus. 2017. *Medicaid and social determinants of health: Adjusting payment and measuring health outcomes.* Health Management Associates. https://www.healthmanagement.com/wp-content/uploads/SHVS_SocialDeterminants_HMA_July2017.pdf (accessed May 26, 2019).

Brewster, A. L., S. Kunkel, J. Straker, and L. A. Curry. 2018. Cross-sectoral partnerships by area agencies on aging: Associations with health care use and spending. *Health Affairs (Millwood)* 37(1):15–21.

Burns, A., and P. Essing. 2018. *Integrating psychosocial risk factors into ongoing care.* Advisory Board. https://www.advisory.com/-/media/Advisory-com/Research/PHA/Research-Briefings/2018/PHA-Psychosocial%20Risk%20Factors%20Brief.pdf (accessed May 26, 2019).

Byhoff, E., E. H. De Marchis, D. Hessler, C. Fichtenberg, N. Adler, A. J. Cohen, K. M. Doran, S. Ettinger de Cuba, E. W. Fleegler, N. Gavin, A. G. Huebschmann, S. T. Lindau, E. L. Tung, M. Raven, S. Jepson, W. Johnson, A. L. Olson, M. Sandel, R. S. Sheward, and L. M. Gottleib. In press. Part II: A qualitative study of social risk screening acceptability in patients and caregivers. *American Journal of Preventive Medicine.*

Cartier, Y., M. Pantell, E. De Marchis, and L. Gottlieb. 2019. *National surveys gauging the prevalence of social care-related activities in the health care sector.* https://sirenetwork.ucsf.edu/tools-resources/mmi/national-surveys-gauging-prevalence-social-care-related-activities-health-care (accessed February 25, 2019).

Chaiyachati, K. H., R. A. Hubbard, A. Yeager, B. Mugo, J. A. Shea, R. Rosin, and D. Grande. 2018. Rideshare-based medical transportation for Medicaid patients and primary care show rates: A difference-in-difference analysis of a pilot program. *Journal of General Internal Medicine* 33(6):863–868.

Chicago Community Loan Fund. 2018. Chicago neighborhood pilot launches workforce services component. https://cclfchicago.org/news/about-us/chicago-neighborhood-rebuild-pilot-launches-workforce-services-component (accessed August 4, 2019).

Chinman, M., R. S. Oberman, B. H. Hanusa, A. N. Cohen, M. P. Salyers, E. W. Twamley, and A. S. Young. 2015. A cluster randomized trial of adding peer specialists to intensive case management teams in the Veterans Health Administration. *Journal of Behavioral Health Services & Research* 42(1):109–121.

CMS (Centers for Medicare & Medicaid Services). 2019. *Accountable health communities model.* https://innovation.cms.gov/initiatives/ahcm (accessed May 26, 2019).

Commonwealth of Massachusetts. 2017. *FAQs for MassHealth's 2017 payment model.* https://www.mass.gov/files/documents/2017/11/07/social-determinants-of-health-faq.pdf (accessed February 5, 2019).

Community Development Financial Insitutions Coalition Report. 2019. http://cdfi.org/wp-content/uploads/2019/03/2019-CDFI-Report-Complete-FINAL.pdf (accessed August 4, 2019).

Crumley, D., and P.-W. Marlise. 2018. *Addressing social determinants of health through Medicaid accountable care organizations.* CHCS Blog: Center for Health Care Strategies. https://www.chcs.org/addressing-social-determinants-health-medicaid-accountable-care-organizations (accessed May 26, 2019).

Dale, J., I. O. Caramlau, A. Lindenmeyer, and S. M. Williams. 2008. Peer support telephone calls for improving health. *Cochrane Database of Systematic Reviews* (4):CD006903.

De Milto, L., and M. Nakashian. 2016. *Using social determinants of health data to improve health care and health: A learning report.* Robert Wood Johnson Foundation. https://www.rwjf.org/en/library/research/2016/04/using-social-determinants-of-health-data-to-improve-health-care-.html (accessed May 26, 2019).

DeSilvey, S., A. Ashbrook, R. Sheward, H. Hartline-Grafton, S. Ettinger de Cuba, and L. Gottlieb. 2018. *An overview of food insecurity coding in health care settings: Existing and emerging opportunities.* Boston, MA: Hunger Vital Sign National Community of Practice. http://www.frac.org/wp-content/uploads/Overview_of_Food_Insecurity_Coding_Report_Final-1.pdf (accessed May 26, 2019).

Dzau, V. J., M. McClellan, J. M. McGinnis, and E. M. Finkelman (eds.). 2017. *Vital directions for health & health care: An initiative of the National Academy of Medicine.* Washington, DC: National Academy of Medicine.

East Baltimore Development Inc. 2010. *About.* http://ebdi.org/about (accessed February 8, 2019).

Eckel, R. H., J. M. Jakicic, J. D. Ard, J. M. de Jesus, N. H. Miller, V. S. Hubbard, I. M. Lee, A. H. Lichtenstein, C. M. Loria, B. E. Millen, C. A. Nonas, F. M. Sacks, S. C. Smith, L. P. Svetkey, T. A. Wadden, and S. Z. Yanovski. 2014. 2013 AHA/ACC guideline on lifestyle management to reduce cardiovascular risk. *Circulation* 129(25 Suppl 2):S76–S99.

Fabbre, V. D., A. S. Buffington, S. J. Altfeld, G. E. Shier, and R. L. Golden. 2011. Social work and transitions of care: Observations from an intervention for older adults. *Journal of Gerontological Social Work* 54(6):615–626.

Feinberg, A. T., J. R. Slotkin, A. Hess, and A. R. Erskine. 2017. *How Geisinger treats diabetes by giving away free, healthy food.* https://hbr.org/2017/10/how-geisinger-treats-diabetes-by-giving-away-free-healthy-food (accessed March 25, 2019).

Felland, L. E., C. S. Lesser, A. B. Staiti, A. Katz, and P. Lichiello. 2003. The resilience of the health care safety net, 1996–2001. *Health Services Research* 38(1 Pt. 2):489–502.

Fleegler, E. W., T. A. Lieu, P. H. Wise, and S. Muret-Wagstaff. 2007. Families' health-related social problems and missed referral opportunities. *Pediatrics* 119(6):e1332–e1341.

Ford-Gilboe, M., C. Herbert, B. E. Jackson, J. G. Lavoie, B. Pauly, N. A. Perrin, V. Smye, C. Varcoe, B. Wallace, N. C. Wathen, S. T. Wong, and A. J. Browne. 2018. How equity-oriented health care affects health: Key mechanisms and implications for primary health care practice and policy. *Milbank Quarterly* 96(4):635–671.

Fraser, M. W., B. M. Lombardi, S. Wu, L. de Saxe Zerden, E. L. Richman, and E. P. Fraher. 2018. Integrated primary care and social work: A systematic review. *Journal of the Society for Social Work and Research* 9(2):175–215.

Garg, A. X., N. K. Adhikari, H. McDonald, M. P. Rosas-Arellano, P. J. Devereaux, J. Beyene, J. Sam, and R. B. Haynes. 2005. Effects of computerized clinical decision support systems on practitioner performance and patient outcomes: A systematic review. *JAMA* 293(10):1223–1238.

Garg, A., R. Boynton-Jarrett, and P. H. Dworkin. 2016. Avoiding the unintended consequences of screening for social determinants of health. *JAMA* 316(8):813–814.

Gaskin, D. J., R. McCleary, and R. J. Thorpe. 2018. The Maryland Health Enterprise Zone Initiative reduced hospital cost and utilization in underserved communities *Determinants of Health* 37(10):1546–1554.

Gehlert, S., S. Collins, R. Golden, and P. Horn. 2015. Social work participation in accountable care organizations under the Patient Protection and Affordable Care Act. *Health & Social Work* 40(4):E142–E147.

Gottlieb, L. M., and H. Alderwick. 2019. Integrating social and medical care: Could it worsen health and increase inequity? *Annals of Family Medicine* 17(1):77–81.

Gottlieb, L., C. Fichtenberg, and N. Adler. 2017a. *Introducing the Social Interventions Research and Evaluation Network..* Social Interventions Research and Evaluation Network. http://sirenetwork.ucsf.edu/sites/sirenetwork.ucsf.edu/files/SIREN%20Issue%20Brief.pdf (accessed May 26, 2019).

Gottlieb, L. M., H. Wing, and N. E. Adler. 2017b. A systematic review of interventions on patients' social and economic needs. *American Journal of Preventative Medicine* 53(5):719–729.

Gunderson, J. M., M. L. Wieland, O. Quirindongo-Cedeno, G. B. Asiedu, J. L. Ridgeway, M. W. O'Brien, T. M. Nelson, R. Buzard, C. Campbell, and J. W. Njeru. 2018. Community health workers as an extension of care coordination in primary care: A community-based cosupervisory model. *Journal of Ambulatory Care Management* 41(4):333–340.

Hager, E. R., A. M. Quigg, M. M. Black, S. M. Coleman, T. Heeren, R. Rose-Jacobs, J. T. Cook, S. A. Ettinger de Cuba, P. H. Casey, M. Chilton, D. B. Cutts, A. F. Meyers, and D. A. Frank. 2010. Development and validity of a 2-item screen to identify families at risk for food insecurity. *Pediatrics* 126(1):e26–e32.

Hannigan, B., and M. Coffey. 2011. Where the wicked problems are: The case of mental health. *Health Policy* 101(3):220–227.

Harkavy, I. 2016. Engaging urban universities as anchor institutions for health equity. *American Journal of Public Health* 106(12):2155–2157.

Healthcare Anchor Network. 2019. *About the healthcare anchor network*. https://www.healthcareanchor.network/about.html (accessed May 24, 2019).

Helfrich, C. D., P. W. Sylling, R. C. Gale, D. C. Mohr, S. E. Stockdale, S. Joos, E. J. Brown, D. Grembowski, S. M. Asch, S. D. Fihn, K. M. Nelson, and L. S. Meredith. 2016. The facilitators and barriers associated with implementation of a patient-centered medical home in VHA. *Implementation Science* 11:24.

Holley, J. L., C. DeVore, T. Obrero, and L. Noland. 2006. Managing homeless dialysis patients. *Nephrology News & Issues* 20(1):49–50, 52–53.

Institute for Alternative Futures. 2012. *Community health centers leveraging the social determinants of health*. http://www.altfutures.org/wp-content/uploads/2016/04/2012_Report_Community-Health-Centers-Leveraging-the-Social-Determinants-of-Health.pdf (accessed May 23, 2019).

IOM (Institute of Medicine). 2012. *An integrated framework for assessing the value of community-based prevention*. Washington, DC: The National Academies Press.

Jensen, M. D., D. H. Ryan, C. M. Apovian, J. D. Ard, A. G. Comuzzie, K. A. Donato, F. B. Hu, V. S. Hubbard, J. M. Jakicic, R. F. Kushner, C. M. Loria, B. E. Millen, C. A. Nonas, F. X. Pi-Sunyer, J. Stevens, V. J. Stevens, T. A. Wadden, B. M. Wolfe, and S. Z. Yanovski. 2014. 2013 AHA/ACC/TOS guideline for the management of overweight and obesity in adults. *Circulation* 129(25 Suppl 2):S102–S138.

JHU (John Hopkins University). 2019. *Homewood Community Partners Initiative*. https://president.jhu.edu/anchor-initiatives/homewood-community-partners-initiative (accessed February 8, 2019).

Kangovi, S., K. Kellom, C. Sha, S. Johnson, C. Chanton, T. Carter, J. A. Long, and D. Grande. 2015. Perceptions of high-risk patients and their providers on the patient-centered medical home. *Journal of Ambulatory Care Management* 38(2):134–143.

Kangovi, S., N. M. Mitra, L. Norton, R. Harte, X. Zhao, T. Carter, D. Grande, and J. A. Long. 2018. Effect of community health worker support on clinical outcomes of low-income patients across primary care facilities: A randomized clinical trial. *JAMA Internal Medicine* 178(12):1635–1643.

Knowles, M. 2018. *Henry Ford Health partners with SPLT, Lyft to get patients to appointment*. https://www.beckershospitalreview.com/patient-flow/henry-ford-health-partners-with-splt-lyft-to-get-patients-to-appointments.html (accessed February 8, 2019).

Ku, L., and G. Flores. 2005. Pay now or pay later: Providing interpreter services in health care. *Health Affairs (Millwood)* 24(2):435–444.

Levinson, W., R. Gorawara-Bhat, and J. Lamb. 2000. A study of patient clues and physician responses in primary care and surgical setting. *JAMA* 284(8):1021–1027.

Lewis, J. H., K. Whelihan, I. Navarro, and K. R. Boyle. 2016. Community health center provider ability to identify, treat, and account for the social determinants of health: A card study. *BMC Family Practice* 17:121.

Lindau, S. T., J. Makelarski, E. Abramsohn, D. G. Beiser, V. Escamilla, J. Jerome, D. Johnson, A. N. Kho, K. K. Lee, T. Long, and D. C. Miller. 2016. CommunityRx: A population health improvement innovation that connects clinics to communities. *Health Affairs (Millwood)* 35(11):2020–2029.

Long, P., M. Abrams, A. Milstein, G. Anderson, K. Lewis Apton, M. Lund Dahlberg, and D. Whicher (eds.). 2017. *Effective care for high-need patients: Opportunities for improving outcomes, value, and health*. Washington, DC: National Academy of Medicine.

Lukens, E. P., and W. R. McFarlane. 2004. Psychoeducation as evidence-based practice: Considerations for practice, research, and policy. *Brief Treatment and Crisis Intervention* 4(3):205–225.

Martin, J., A. Martin, C. Schultz, and M. Sandel. 2015. *Embedding civil legal aid services in care for high-utilizing patients using medical–legal partnership.* Health Affairs blog. https://www.healthaffairs.org/do/10.1377/hblog20150422.047143/full (accessed May 26, 2019).

Martinez, M. 2018. *Ford partners with Beaumont Health on medical transport service.* https://www.crainsdetroit.com/article/20180418/news/658481/ford-partners-with-beaumont-health-on-medical-transport-service (accessed February 8, 2019).

MassHealth. 2018a. *MassHealth accountable care organizations (ACOs).* https://massdocs-digital-mass-gov.s3.amazonaws.com/s3fs-public/2018/MassHealth%2520ACO%2520One-Pager_0.pdf?HQAkdYxhMJTUv2ZGcn9IODj0Dm72uVJV (accessed May 26, 2019).

MassHealth. 2018b. *MassHealth flexible services program.* https://www.mass.gov/files/documents/2018/11/14/MassHealth%20Flexible%20Services%20One%20Pager.pdf (accessed May 26, 2019).

Mays, G. P., C. B. Mamaril, and L. R. Timsina. 2016. Preventable death rates fell where communities expanded population health activities through multisector networks. *Health Affairs (Millwood)* 35(11):2005–2013.

McGinnis, T., M. Crawford, and S. A. Somers. 2014. A state policy framework for integrating health and social services. *Issue Brief (Commonwealth Fund)* 14:1–9.

Miller, W. R., and S. Rollnick. 2012. *Motivational interviewing: Helping people change, 3rd ed.* New York: Guilford Press.

NASDOH (National Alliance to Impact the Social Determinants of Health). 2019. *Who we are.* http://www.nasdoh.org (accessed March 25, 2019).

NASEM (National Academies of Sciences, Engineering, and Medicine). 2016. *Systems practices for the care of socially at-risk populations.* Washington, DC: The National Academies Press.

Navathe, A. S., F. Zhong, V. J. Lei, F. Y. Chang, M. Sordo, M. Topaz, S. B. Navathe, R. A. Rocha, and L. Zhou. 2018. Hospital readmission and social risk factors identified from physician notes. *Health Services Research* 53(2):1110–1136.

NEJM Catalyst. 2017. *What is patient-centered care?* January 1. https://catalyst.nejm.org/what-is-patient-centered-care (accessed May 26, 2019).

Ockene, J. K., E. A. Edgerton, S. M. Teutsch, L. N. Marion, T. Miller, J. L. Genevro, C. J. Loveland-Cherry, J. E. Fielding, and P. A. Briss. 2007. Integrating evidence-based clinical and community strategies to improve health. *American Journal of Preventative Medicine* 32(3):244–252.

Palakshappa, D., S. Doupnik, A. Vasan, S. Khan, L. Seifu, C. Feudtner, and A. G. Fiks. 2017. Suburban families' experience with food insecurity screening in primary care practices. *Pediatrics* 140(1):e20170320.

Plough, A. L. 2015. *Measuring what matters: Introducing a new action framework.* Robert Wood Johnson Foundation Culture of Health Blog. https://www.rwjf.org/en/blog/2015/11/measuring_what_matte.html (accessed May 26, 2019).

Podymow, T., and J. Turnbull. 2013. Management of chronic kidney disease and dialysis in homeless persons. *Kidney International Supplements (2011)* 3(2):230–235.

Primm, B. J., L. Perez, G. C. Dennis, L. Benjamin, H. W. Clark, K. Keough, W. D. Leak, R. Payne, D. Smith, and L. W. Sullivan. 2004. Managing pain: The challenge in underserved populations: Appropriate use versus abuse and diversion. *Journal of the National Medical Assocation* 96(9):1152–1161.

Repper, J., and T. Carter. 2011. A review of the literature on peer support in mental health services. *Journal of Mental Health* 20(4):392–411.

Rizzo, V. M., and J. M. Rowe. 2016. Studies of the cost-effectiveness of social work services in aging: An updated review of the literature. *Research on Social Work Practice* 26(6):609–621.

Rizzo, V. M., J. M. Rowe, G. Shier Kricke, K. Krajci, and R. Golden. 2016. AIMS: A care coordination model to improve patient health outcomes. *Health & Social Work* 41(3):191–195.

Rowe, J., V. Rizzo, D. Guthrie, M. Vail, S. Kang, and R. Golden. 2019. The electronic health record: Documenting the unique contributions of social workers. *Health & Social Work* 44(2):123–128. doi: 10.1093/hsw/hlz006.

Rowe, J., V. Rizzo, S. Kang, R. Kukowski, M. Newman, B. Ewald, and R. Golden. In press. Time contribution of social workers in care management: Value for older adults. *Professional Case Management*.

RUMC (Rush University Medical Center). 2017. *Rush to make $6 million in impact investments*. https://www.rush.edu/news/press-releases/rush-makes-first-impact-investment?mc_cid=2f88162828&mc_eid=98430b86a6 (accessed April 12, 2019).

Salzer, M., E. Schwenk, and E. Brusilovskiy. 2010. Certified peer specialist roles and activities: Results from a national survey *Psychiatric Services* 61(5):520–523.

Sambare, T., L. Uhler, and K. J. Bozic. 2017. Shared decision making: Time to get personal. *NEJM Catalyst*, October 12. https://catalyst.nejm.org/shared-decision-making (accessed April 10, 2019).

Schoenthaler, A., G. J. Knafl, K. Fiscella, and G. Ogedegbe. 2017. Addressing the social needs of hypertensive patients: The role of patient–provider communication as a predictor of medication adherence. *Circulation: Cardiovascular Quality and Outcomes* 10(9):e003659.

Schrage, D. 2018. *Building partnerships with primary care to become a hub for service delivery for older adults in our community*. Aging and Disability Business Institute blog, June 28. https://www.aginganddisabilitybusinessinstitute.org/building-partnerships-with-primary-care-to-become-a-hub-for-service-delivery-for-older-adults-in-our-community (accessed May 26, 2019).

Seligman, H. K., A. F. Bolger, D. Guzman, A. Lopez, and K. Bibbins-Domingo. 2014. Exhaustion of food budgets at month's end and hospital admissions for hypoglycemia. *Health Affairs (Millwood)* 33(1):116–123.

Stanhope, V., and S. Straussner. 2017. *Social work and integrated health care*. New York: Oxford University Press.

Steiner, J. F., J. L. Adams, D. Clausen, K. M. Clift, A. Millan, C. L. Nau, D. Roblin, J. A. Schmittdiel, and E. B. Schroeder. 2018. *Predictive Models for Social Determinants of Health in KP Members and Communities: An Issue Brief from Kaiser Permanente's Social Needs Network for Evaluation and Translation (SONNET)*. Kaiser Permanente SONNET and Kaiser Permanente Community Health, September 2018.

Stone, N. J., J. G. Robinson, A. H. Lichtenstein, C. N. Bairey Merz, C. B. Blum, R. H. Eckel, A. C. Goldberg, D. Gordon, D. Levy, D. M. Lloyd-Jones, P. McBride, J. S. Schwartz, S. T. Shero, S. C. Smith, Jr., K. Watson, P. W. Wilson, K. M. Eddleman, N. M. Jarrett, K. LaBresh, L. Nevo, J. Wnek, J. L. Anderson, J. L. Halperin, N. M. Albert, B. Bozkurt, R. G. Brindis, L. H. Curtis, D. DeMets, J. S. Hochman, R. J. Kovacs, E. M. Ohman, S. J. Pressler, F. W. Sellke, W. K. Shen, S. C. Smith, Jr., G. F. Tomaselli, and American College of Cardiology/American Heart Association Task Force on Practice Guidelines. 2014. 2013 ACC/AHA guideline on the treatment of blood cholesterol to reduce atherosclerotic cardiovascular risk in adults: A report of the American College of Cardiology/American Heart Association Task Force on Practice Guidelines. *Circulation* 129(25 Suppl 2):S1–S45.

Swavely, D., V. Whyte, J. F. Steiner, and S. L. Freeman. 2018. Complexities of addressing food insecurity in an urban population. *Population Health Management* 22(4):300–307.

Tong, S. T., W. R. Liaw, P. Lail Kashiri, J. Pecsok, J. Rozman, A. Bazemore, and A. H. Kirst. 2018. Clinician experiences with screening for social needs in primary care. *Journal of the American Board of Family Medicine* 31(3):351–363.

Torres, J. M., J. Lawlor, J. D. Colvin, M. R. Sills, J. L. Bettenhausen, A. Davidson, G. J. Cutler, M. Hall, and L. M. Gottlieb. 2017. ICD social codes: An underutilized resource for tracking social needs. *Medical Care* 55(9):810–816.

Towe, V. L., L. Leviton, A. Chandra, J. C. Sloan, M. Tait, and T. Orleans. 2016. Cross-sector collaborations and partnerships: Essential ingredients to help shape health and well-being. *Health Affairs (Millwood)* 35(11):1964–1969.

Ubhayakar, S., M. Capeless, R. Owens, K. Snorrason, and D. Zuckerman. 2017. *Anchor Mission playbook.* Chicago: Rush University Medical Center. https://www.rush.edu/sites/default/files/anchor-mission-playbook.pdf (accessed May 26, 2019).

UCSF (University of California, San Francisco). 2019. *SIREN: Social Needs Screening Tools Comparison Table (Pediatric Settings).* http://sirenetwork.ucsf.edu/tools-resources/mmi/screening-tools-comparison/peds (accessed May 10, 2019).

UnitedHealth Group. 2013. *UnitedHealth Group, Minnesota Equity Fund, and community leaders celebrate opening of affordable-housing community in Ramsey.* November 14. https://www.unitedhealthgroup.com/newsroom/2013/1114mnaffordablehousing.html (accessed February 8, 2019).

VA (U.S. Department of Veterans Affairs). 2019. *VA research on homelessness.* https://www.research.va.gov/topics/homelessness.cfm (accessed April 12, 2019).

Vickery, K. D., N. D. Shippee, J. Menk, R. Owen, D. M. Vock, P. Bodurtha, D. Soderlund, R. A. Hayward, M. M. Davis, J. Connett, and M. Linzer. 2018. Integrated, accountable care for Medicaid expansion enrollees: A comparative evaluation of Hennepin Health. *Medical Care Research and Review,* May 1 [Epub ahead of print].

Waite, R. 2018. *Synergy: Bridging the gap between intentionality and actuality: Building resilience and wellbeing through partnership, courage, connection and compassion.* Presentation to the Committee on Integrating Social Needs Care into the Delivery of Health Care to Improve the Nation's Health, September 24, 2018, Washington, DC.

Wasserman, M., M. R. Renfrew, A. R. Green, L. Lopez, A. Tan-McGrory, C. Brach, and J. R. Betancourt. 2014. Identifying and preventing medical errors in patients with limited English proficiency: Key findings and tools for the field. *Journal of Healthcare Quality* 36(3):5–16.

Weiner, S., and A. Schwartz. 2016. *Listening for what matters: Avoiding contextual errors in health care.* New York: Oxford University Press.

Weiner, S. J., A. Schwartz, F. Weaver, J. Goldberg, R. Yudkowsky, G. Sharma, A. Binns-Calvey, B. Preyss, M. M. Schapira, S. D. Persell, E. Jacobs, and R. I. Abrams. 2010. Contextual errors and failures in individualizing patient care. *Annals of Internal Medicine* 153(2):69–75.

3

A Workforce to Integrate Social Care into Health Care Delivery

Workforce availability and the competence of workers to serve the needs of complex vulnerable populations and address adverse social determinants of health (SDOH) is not a new subject for the National Academies of Sciences, Engineering, and Medicine (the National Academies). Among the National Academies reports that have addressed this topic are *Retooling for an Aging America: Building the Health Care Workforce* (IOM, 2008), *The Mental Health and Substance Use Workforce for Older Adults: In Whose Hands?* (IOM, 2012), *Measuring the Impact of Interprofessional Education on Collaborative Practice and Patient Outcomes* (IOM, 2015), *A Framework for Educating Health Professionals to Address the Social Determinants of Health* (NASEM, 2016a), *Strengthening the Workforce to Support Community Living and Participation for Older Adults and Individuals with Disabilities* (NASEM, 2017), and *Effective Care for High-Need Patients: Opportunities for Improving Outcomes, Value, and Health* (Long et al., 2017). In addition, reports produced by the U.S. Department of Health and Human Services, such as *Addressing the Social Determinants of Health: The Role of Health Professions Education* (Committee on Training in Primary Care Medicine and Dentistry, 2016), shed light on the critical issues of the role of the workforce in addressing social determinants and provide recommendations for improvement. Collectively, these reports establish the foundation required to discuss how to best prepare and support a workforce to address the social needs of populations as one component of health care delivery.

Evidence linking the SDOH with a population's health status and health care costs has led to efforts to redesign health care and to better link the provision of health care with the provision of social services in ways that address the factors that contribute to the poor health of patients and communities. Chapter 2 identified five complementary activities that health care systems can adopt in order to strengthen social care integration: awareness, adjustment, assistance, alignment, and advocacy. Implementing and sustaining efforts within each of the five activities will require making systems-level changes, including the development of a well-trained workforce with defined roles, innovations in data and digital tools, and new financing models. This chapter focuses on the necessary elements of a workforce that will have the capability and capacity to improve social care within these five activities.

THE PROMISE OF INTERPROFESSIONAL TEAMS IN IMPROVING SOCIAL CARE

There is a consensus among agencies and organizations as well as among educators and clinicians that addressing the adverse SDOH is complex and requires an interprofessional team (NASEM, 2016b). Teamwork in health care has been associated with improvements in knowledge, practice, and such outcomes as quality, cost reduction, and job satisfaction (Medves et al., 2010). Effective collaboration among teams requires explicitly defined tasks and goals, clear and meaningful roles for each individual, and systematic guidelines to assist practitioner in their decision making. The use of in-person and technology-based mechanisms to minimize gaps in care and to avoid duplication of services is important since many team members may be working remotely from one another. The processes that are important in optimizing the functioning of a team include collaboration and coordination, the pooling of resources, and role blurring, which is defined as creating a shared body of knowledge and skills among team members so that various elements of professionals' roles can be taken on by others, if necessary (Sims et al., 2015).

Tackling the complex social needs of patients and families requires collaboration, both on the team and outside of the traditional health care sector, such as on the staffs of social service and public health agencies and community-based organizations.[1] As such, the list of individuals who may be considered team members has been expanding. For example, lawyers have become critical team members for addressing legal matters related to housing and other social factors among patients in community

[1] As detailed below, types of workers who provide social care can include nurses; physicians; social workers; community health workers; social service navigators, aides, assistants, and trained volunteers; home health aides; personal care aides; family caregivers; case managers; gerontologists; lawyers; and others.

health centers (Regenstein et al., 2018). As more organizations and payers address social needs, competencies should be established to ensure that interprofessional teams are equipped to work together optimally within the complex and shifting landscape of social care. The competencies established for behavioral and primary care workers are an example of how competencies can be used for interprofessional teams (Hoge et al., 2014).

How effectively interprofessional teams are able to carry out their day-to-day work is dependent on several factors that, if not taken into account, can hamper integration and collaboration among team members. One such important factor is role clarity—that is, how well team members know their own and the other's roles and responsibilities (Ambrose-Miller and Ashcroft, 2016; Sims et al., 2015). Social needs are best addressed when members of the interprofessional team understand the role that each team member plays, both directly and indirectly, in the awareness, adjustment, assistance, alignment, and advocacy activities described in Chapter 2. Team members should understand the knowledge, skills, and competencies that each member brings, and each member should be able to work at the full scope of his or her knowledge, skills, and competencies (Glaser and Suter, 2016; Lombardi et al., 2017; Sims et al., 2015). Other factors aiding in the effective functioning of interprofessional teams include allowing team members to maintain their professional identities, particularly in the case of social care workers who work within health care (Garfield and Kangovi, 2019), and addressing issues related to power dynamics among team members (Ambrose-Miller and Ashcroft, 2016). Attributes of successful interprofessional teams include a commitment by staff members to work in a team environment, communication among the staff, and the ability of staff members to come up with creative ways to conduct their work (Molyneux, 2001). According to Sims and colleagues

> Teams are complex entities influenced by human and organizations factors and the field of health they operate in. This makes teamworking highly variable and context dependent, which means that different teams will succeed in different situations depending upon the processes, participants, and context in which they are based. (Sims et al., 2015, p. 20)

Interprofessional education—defined as "when students from two or more professions learn about, from, and with each other to enable effective collaboration and improve health outcomes" (WHO, 2010a, p. 7)—is an important approach to developing effective interprofessional teams that can address the integration of social care into health care. Recommendations from both the Institute of Medicine's (IOM's) *Health Professions Education: A Bridge to Quality* report and the Interprofessional Education Collaborative have called for curriculum and learning activities designed to develop competencies among health care and social service professionals in the delivery of patient-centered team care (IOM, 2003a; IPEC, 2011).

More educational institutions are developing and providing core curricula to health care and social service providers. Some professions have embraced the need for interprofessional team collaboration to assure that their workers are equipped with the skills, knowledge, and abilities necessary to provide effective team care and to address the social needs of patient populations. The most effective interprofessional education programs combine coursework with clinical and service learning experiences in the community (Greer et al., 2018; Siegel et al., 2018; Zomorodi et al., 2018). For example, physicians accompanying a social worker on home visits typically come away with a new appreciation for how the social needs that were identified could compromise the care plan they had in mind (Fulmer et al., 2004).

The pathway from initial education to practice behaviors is complex (IOM, 2015) (see Figure 3-1). In considering how best to develop a health

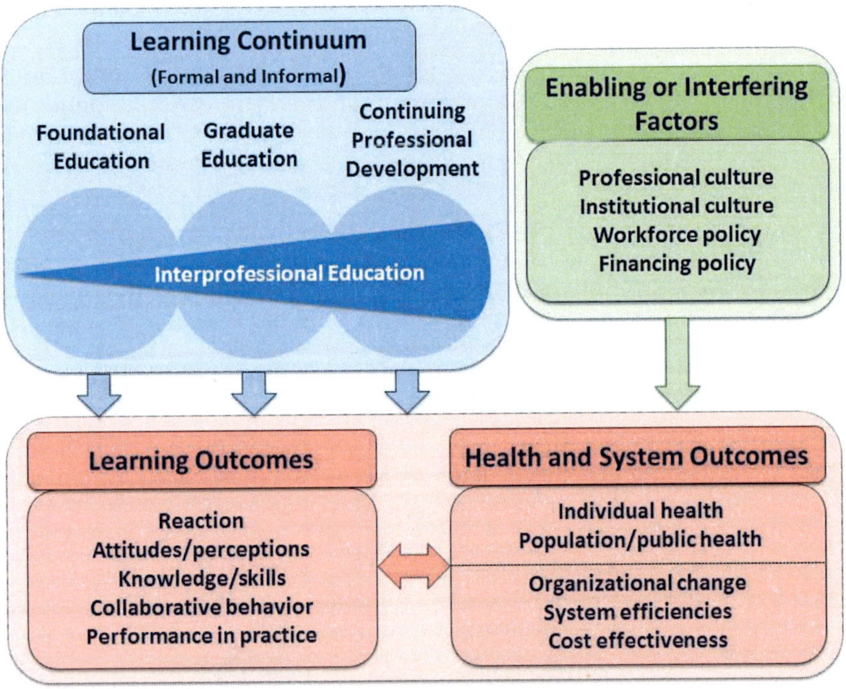

FIGURE 3-1 The interprofessional learning continuum model.
NOTE: For this model, "graduate education" encompasses any advanced formal or supervised health professions training taking place between the completion of foundational education and entry into unsupervised practice.
SOURCE: IOM, 2015.

care workforce that understands and can take into account social factors, it is important to recognize that a health worker's ability to address social needs can be affected by various external factors. Among the factors that can influence the training of health care workers and their delivery of care are the professional and institutional cultures in which they train and work as well as various workforce and financial policies. The conceptual model shown in Figure 3-1, which assumes interprofessional education to be the gold standard for health and social service training, includes the education-to-practice continuum and a broad array of learning, health, and system outcomes, and it shows the major enabling and interfering factors that affect the education-to-practice pathway. This model was put forth with the understanding that it requires empirical testing and that it may have to be adapted to the particular settings in which it is applied.

The development and implementation of effective interprofessional team training programs face a number of challenges. For example, a national evaluation of The John A. Hartford Foundation's Geriatric Interdisciplinary Team Training program found that the attitudinal and cultural traditions of the different health professions faculty and students (usually split along disciplinary lines) are important obstacles to creating an optimal interdisciplinary team training experience (Reuben et al., 2004). In general, physician trainees participated least enthusiastically in geriatric interdisciplinary team training. Among the other challenges to establishing effective interprofessional team training programs are various logistical issues, such as dealing with differences in educational calendars among the different professions and class schedules. At the heart of the challenge in installing team-based approaches as a key part of professional education is what Frenk and colleagues referred to as "tribalism of the professions—that is, the tendency for the various professions to act in isolation from or even in competition with each other" (Frenk et al., 2010, p. 1923).

THE TRADITIONAL HEALTH CARE WORKFORCE

As noted above, effectively addressing people's complex social needs requires that workers within the traditional health care system collaborate with workers from outside of it, such as the staff of social service and public health agencies and community-based organizations. This team approach is not one size fits all. The composition of teams can vary depending on such factors as the available resources (e.g., human, technological, and financial resources), the circumstances (e.g., urban versus rural location), and importantly, which of the five activities (awareness, adjustment, assistance, alignment, and advocacy) is being addressed. An awareness of the SDOH and social care is essential. Just as established competencies and training measures ensure that professionals within the social care landscape can work together and communicate effectively, it is crucial that traditional health care workers know about social care. Health professional organizations are increasingly interested in adding curricular content on addressing the SDOH to health professional education (HRSA, 2016). The competencies related to the SDOH include cultural humility, reflection, advocacy, cultural competency, partnership skills, patient communication, and empathy.

The nursing profession has long focused on the social needs of people and communities (Buhler-Wilkerson, 1993; Fee and Garofalo, 2010). Acute care nurses are expected to also address the psychosocial needs of patients, whether through referrals to social workers or care managers or as part of the discharge planning process. Some nurses are care managers and have great involvement in addressing social needs within health care delivery. Home care nurses assess patients' and families' social needs and may refer patients who have complex social needs to social workers. Nurses in home visitation programs for high-risk mothers and children, such as the Nurse-Family Partnership, address social supports, employment, education, and various other aspects of the mothers' lives such as how to reduce contact with the criminal justice system. These activities are important to short- and long-term maternal and child outcomes (Olds et al., 2007; Williams et al., 2008). Other examples of nurse-designed models of care that successfully integrate the social needs of individuals and families have been documented in a 2018 RAND report (Martsolf et al., 2017).

In its 2008 report *The Essentials of Baccalaureate Education for Professional Nursing Practice*, the American Association of Colleges of Nursing (AACN) defined the essentials of a baccalaureate education in nursing, noting that programs are expected to educate graduates who can "apply knowledge of social and cultural factors to the care of diverse populations" (AACN, 2008, p. 12) and "facilitate patient-centered transitions of care, including discharge planning and ensuring the caregiver's knowledge of care requirements to promote safe care" (AACN, 2008, p. 31). The AACN commissioned a "visioning" task force for defining the future of nursing education. The resulting vision includes educating nurses about the SDOH, and this is expected to be included in the next version of *The Essentials of Baccalaureate Education for Professional Nursing Practice*.[2] The National League for Nursing intends to undertake similar work to include the SDOH and social care in its recommendations for nursing curricula.[3]

[2] Personal communication, Deborah Trautman, American Association of Colleges of Nursing, October 17, 2018.

[3] Personal communication, Beverly Malone, National League for Nursing, October 1, 2018.

Physicians, particularly those working in primary care (including internal medicine, pediatrics, geriatrics, and family medicine) are increasingly expected to recognize the role of social risk factors and social needs in the prevention and treatment of illness and disability. No systematic studies have been done, however, to determine the prevalence of physicians' awareness of or engagement in social care integration or what types of physicians may use which types of activities more frequently.

For those physicians who have completed medical school and are in postgraduate training, the Accreditation Council for Graduate Medical Education has identified several competencies that support physician involvement in addressing patients' social needs. Some of the competencies are related to awareness activities, such as being able to communicate effectively with patients, families, and the public, as appropriate, across a broad range of socioeconomic and cultural backgrounds. Others of the competencies are related to assistance activities, such as the ability to work in interprofessional teams to enhance patient safety and improve patient care quality; having sensitivity and responsiveness to a diverse patient population, including patients diverse in gender, age, culture, race, religion, disabilities, and sexual orientation; and being able to work effectively as members or leaders of a health care team or other professional group (ACGME/ABFM, 2015; Cate, 2013; Leipzig et al., 2014; Parks et al., 2014).

When physician residency programs do include content on the SDOH, it is largely didactic and provided in short or one-time sessions (Gard et al., 2018). Some residency programs include more extensive content on the SDOH; for example, Florida International University's Herbert Wertheim College of Medicine has a service-learning experience in the community with an interprofessional team of students (including nursing and public health) that integrates the SDOH, professional teamwork competencies (including nursing and public health), and community collaboration (Greer et al., 2018). There is a growing recognition of the need to include formal education about the SDOH as part of physician training, and some medical schools are calling for a dramatic rethinking of the social mission of medical schools more broadly, including their responsibility to focus educational, research, clinical, and community service efforts on the SDOH, particularly for the communities where they are located (Mullan, 2017). A review of the literature found rising interest in making the SDOH as part of medical education (Doobay-Persaud et al., 2019). Medical education leaders and experts also are supportive of increasing the exposure to the SDOH across the medical education curriculum; doing this, however, will require development of a common curriculum, standardizing teaching methods, and standard approaches to evaluating impact (Mangold et al., 2019).

SOCIAL CARE WORKFORCE

Ideally, all members of an interprofessional team should have a baseline understanding of social care and the SDOH, but that likely will not be sufficient; effectively integrating social care into health care beyond the level of awareness may require developing a workforce with expertise and a scope of work that are specific to social care. The following discussion provides information that should be considered when developing interprofessional teams, including details about the necessary skill sets and the key professions involved with providing social care. Depending on the social needs of a particular population, it may make sense to include other professions on the team beyond those discussed below (e.g., clergy, medical interpreters, or oral health providers). The composition of interprofessional teams will vary depending on the model of care.

Social Workers

There is a long history of professional social workers providing social care within both the health care and social service sectors, and many social workers have expertise in these fields (Gehlert and Browne, 2011). Social workers assess and address the social needs and well-being of people's lives, whether through direct interventions at the micro level (awareness and assistance activities aimed at the individual and family) or through activities at the meso level (adjustment and alignment activities within the health care system) and macro level (alignment and advocacy at the socio-structural level) (Newman et al., 2015; USC, 2019).

Social workers have led efforts to build bridges between the silos of social services and health care through interventions such as care management and transitional care that take advantage of social work expertise in patient and family engagement, assessment, care planning, behavioral health, and systems navigation (Fraser et al., 2018). By speaking the "language" of—and understanding the important roles of—both community and medical providers, social workers can play an important role in ensuring effective collaboration and communication across the care continuum. They also lead community-based organizations that focus on the social needs and well-being of individuals and families in communities (Pecukonis et al., 2013). Medical social workers are directly involved with the health of individuals and work in a variety of settings, typically hospitals, outpatient clinics, community health agencies, social service agencies, skilled nursing facilities, long-term care facilities, hospices, and health insurers' offices.

Professional social workers obtain a baccalaureate or master's degree in social work, and both bachelor's- and master's-level social workers can seek licensure. Master's-degreed social workers can also seek licensure as a clinical social worker as a specialty within the master degree.[4] Licensure requirements vary by state, but typically involve an exam and a minimum amount of clinical hours with supervision by a licensed clinical social worker. Social workers' education and training cover many of the SDOH competencies noted above. For example, the social work profession, through the National Association of Social Workers, has developed a number of specialized standards of practice that focus on the needs for clinical services of special populations or within specific care settings (NASW, 2016). Several of these standards are particularly relevant to social care in health care delivery. One notable standard for clinical social work in social work practice is: "Clinical social workers shall be knowledgeable about community services and make appropriate referrals, as needed" (NASW, 2005, p. 4). A comprehensive set of standards exists for social work practice done within health care settings, including, for example,

> Social workers practicing in health care settings shall advocate for the needs and interests of clients and client support systems and promote system-level change to improve outcomes, access to care, and delivery of services, particularly for marginalized, medically complex, or disadvantaged populations. (NASW, 2016, p. 29)

In the area of practice in interprofessional teams, the standards for social workers in health care settings include, for instance, "Social workers practicing in health care settings shall promote collaboration among health care team members, other colleagues, and organizations to support, enhance, and deliver effective services to clients and client support systems" (NASW, 2016, p. 31).

Community Health Workers

Community health workers (CHWs) provide linkages among health, social services, and the community (APHA, 2019). Often recruited from the communities they serve, CHWs work in health systems, social service agencies, and community-based organizations. There is a growing number of CHWs employed in hospitals and health systems as well (Malcarney et al., 2017). They are engaged in awareness, assistance, and advocacy activities. All but three states have efforts related to integrating CHWs into health care systems (NASHP, 2017).

There is growing evidence of their positive impact on health, particularly for low-income and minority patients. Several outcome studies

[4] This text has been revised since prepublication release.

related to the use of CHWs have been conducted. The Penn Center for Community Health Workers developed and tested the IMPaCT model, a standardized and scalable CHW intervention; two clinical trials have documented the positive effect of the model (Kangovi et al., 2017, 2018). A systematic review of the literature concluded that there is some evidence that the use of CHWs to help care for the chronically ill could reduce the use of health care and costs (Jack et al., 2017). It is important to note, however, that these studies of the role of CHWs in bridging medical and social care did not clearly articulate whether the CHWs' social care was the component of the intervention that actually achieved health outcomes.

Efforts are under way to develop competencies and standardize educational requirements for CHWs (Rosenthal et al., 2016). The North Carolina Community Health Worker Initiative provides technical assistance from CHW experts through the Association of State and Territorial Health Officials with the aims of confirming the roles and competencies of CHWs, standardizing their training and certification, and identifying the infrastructure and policy supports necessary for the effective use of CHWs (NC DHHS, 2019). The global need for such standardization of the CHW role, training, and infrastructure development has been recognized by the World Health Organization (WHO, 2010b).

According to a 2003 IOM report, barriers to the integration of CHWs into health care delivery include inconsistencies in the scope of practice, training, and qualifications; a lack of sustainable funding; and insufficient recognition by other health professionals (IOM, 2003b). Certification has been established in a number of states, but the requirements (both education- and career-wise) vary widely. Training requirements range from 80 hours to 160 hours, with various provisions for "grandfathering" experienced CHWs (CDC, 2016). The lack of universal professional standards has been described as part of the rationale for the establishment of the National Association of Community Health Workers, which launched in April 2019 (NACHW, 2019).

Social Service Navigators, Aides, and Assistants

Social service navigators, aides, and assistants, and also trained volunteers often work outside of the health care sector in awareness, assistance, and advocacy roles in social service agencies and community-based organizations. Examples include housing and transportation experts, people who work at food banks, people who provide employment assistance, outreach and enrollment workers, navigators, and trained volunteers. These workers assist patients and families on a wide range of activities and often help them find and access services in the community. There is currently no national certification or credentialing for social service navigators, aides, and assistants, or for trained volunteers. Requirements for these workers vary by state, but the workers typically must have at least a high school diploma and must complete a brief period of on-the-job training.

Home Health Aides and Personal Care Aides

Within the health care sector, home health aides and personal care aides provide extensive social support services to assist older adults and disabled and post-acute care patients in their homes. These direct care workers have close contact with the country's most disadvantaged patients. Working in the home, they can directly observe a wide variety of their clients' social needs and then provide this information to other members of the care team. They have an important role to play in the assistance activity in providing social care.

Family Caregivers

People who provide care for their family members (family caregivers) are another critical part of the care team and provide assistance to many individuals. Because they spend time in the home, family caregivers, similar to home health aides and personal care aides, have a valuable perspective on the social needs of patients. In 2015 more than 43 million Americans provided unpaid care to high-need individuals, with an estimated 85 percent of them being family members (Family Caregiver Alliance, 2016). These caregivers provide a wide range of services, including complex medical–nursing tasks such as managing multiple medications, providing wound care, and using medical-related monitors; assisting with activities of daily living; transportation; and communicating with and visiting with health care providers (Reinhard et al., 2012).

Case Managers

Case managers (and care managers) work intensively with individuals with complex social needs, whether in the health care system or with social service agencies. An increasing number are certified, as health care organizations and other employers increasingly require certification for hiring or continuing employment (Tahan et al., 2006). Case managers focus on coordinating the health and social care of patients and work within the spheres of awareness, assistance, and advocacy (at the individual level). They can be based in hospitals, at home care agencies, in skilled nursing and rehabilitation facilities, or with community-based organizations. Case managers also are found in social services agencies, such as foster care agencies, child welfare agencies, senior centers, and homeless shelters. Often, the role of case managers is filled by licensed clinical social workers and licensed nurses.

Promising Additional Professions for Improving Social Care

Gerontologists

Gerontology is a discipline that holds promise for addressing the social needs of the older adult population. According to the Academy for Gerontology in Higher Education (AGHE), "gerontologists improve the quality of life and promote the well-being of persons as they age within their families, communities, and societies through research, education, and application of interdisciplinary knowledge of the aging process and aging populations" (AGHE, 2019). Functional health and independence are the goals of care for older adults, and therefore addressing social needs is a component of addressing health care needs. AGHE has identified core and contextual competencies that support the roles of gerontologists in the five categories of activities that promote social care as part of health care delivery (AGHE, 2014).

Gerontology is not well defined in terms of how it relates to social care. Unlike other types of health and social services disciplines, there is no licensure, scope of work, or U.S. Department of Labor recognition for gerontologists. In 2016 the Accreditation for Gerontology Education Council was established to accredit gerontology education programs at the associate, baccalaureate, and master's levels. This is an important step in the development of the profession and will further link the AGHE competencies to gerontology education programs and social care practice. According to the National Association for Professional Gerontologists, certified gerontologists report holding such positions as direct service providers (health and community support services), administrators, chief executive officers, entrepreneurs and business owners, therapists and counselors, resource navigators and information specialists, program directors, professors, researchers, pastors, and geriatricians and other medical doctors.[5] In certain states, organizations employing gerontologists with at least a bachelor's degree can be reimbursed for services specified in the waiver agreement with the Centers for Medicare & Medicaid Services' Home and Community-Based Services Program (California Department of Health Care Services, 2019). These services vary by state, but often include a home- and community-based services wellness assessment and case management services. Because older adults often have

[5] Personal communication, Donna Schaefer, August 29, 2018.

complex medical and social needs, expanding the use of gerontologists in these roles will provide an additional resource for increasing social care.

Lawyers

Lawyers who address the social needs of patients and families are increasingly being used in community-based organizations, including some federally qualified health centers, to assist patients and families with legal matters that can compromise health, such as inadequate housing or a loss of housing. Medical–legal partnerships integrate the unique expertise of lawyers into health care settings in order to help clinicians, social workers, and care managers address the social needs of patients in ways that can reduce many health inequities (Regenstein et al., 2018). There are many different types of lawyers, but one type in particular is relevant to social care: the public interest lawyer.

> Public interest lawyers work for private, nonprofit organizations that provide legal services to disadvantaged people or others who otherwise might not be able to afford legal representation. They generally handle civil cases, such as those having to do with leases, job discrimination, and wage disputes, rather than criminal cases. (BLS, 2019)

Increasing the availability and involvement of public interest lawyers will help in providing social care to the vulnerable populations.

CHALLENGES AND BARRIERS FOR SOCIAL CARE WORKERS

The social care workforce faces a number of challenges and barriers to practice at the individual level, organizational level, and systems level. More information on the workforce challenges related to integrating social care into the delivery of health care is presented in Chapter 6.

Individual worker-level challenges can be divided into several categories: worker health and well-being, including issues related to burnout, violence, and suicide; worker satisfaction, including issues related to compensation, incentives, perceived value, and sense of identity; and negative attitudes regarding the SDOH and "blaming the victim" (Bodenheimer and Sinsky, 2014; Bride, 2007; Eelen et al., 2014; Hart and Warren, 2013; Kim et al., 2018; Martin and Schinke, 1998). These individual-level challenges can be worsened by a lack of organizational capacity to address adverse social conditions, which can exacerbate professional burnout, particularly by affecting providers' self-efficacy (De Marchis et al., 2019; Olayiwola et al., 2018; Pantell et al., 2019).

Organizational-level challenges include issues relating to the hierarchy of leadership of health and social service professionals and the siloed nature of health care and social services (Ellner and Phillips, 2017), role limitations in care settings (La Motte, 2012), issues relating to work and case load assignments, and the orientations and values of educational institutions (NASEM, 2016a).

Systems-level challenges include barriers to reimbursement for certain types of workers (Houston and Mahadevan, 2015; HRSA, 2018a), inadequate numbers of workers, and workforces that are not demographically representative of the populations they serve (Lin et al., 2016; NASEM, 2016a; Warshaw and Bragg, 2014).

Medicare payments and policy have substantially influenced medical and clinical social work. In 1989 the Omnibus Budget Reconciliation Act amended the Social Security Act to include clinical social work services under Medicare Part B covered services, defining clinical social work services as services related to the "diagnosis and treatment of mental illnesses" (summarized in Zarrella, 2005). This change enabled licensed social workers to bill Medicare for individual and group psychotherapy, which contributed to social work becoming the largest behavioral health workforce in the United States (Heisler, 2018; Zarrella, 2005). However, this definition of clinical social work is limiting in that it does not reflect the broad array of services that clinical social workers provide, which creates confusion about social work's scope of practice despite curricula and core competencies that reach beyond behavioral health diagnosis and treatment. As a result, no matter whether they practice independently, as part of a health care organization, or as part of a community-based organization, social workers are defined in Medicare only as mental health providers and not as carrying out other roles such as care managers or the providers of psychoeducation that help patients adapt to a new diagnosis. This means that no matter the practice setting, social workers' work is not adequately captured by Medicare fee-for-service billing options. Importantly, the definition's exclusive focus on behavioral health has largely prevented social workers from using health and behavior assessment and intervention codes for billing, even though it is these codes that reimburse for services that target social factors resulting from or affecting physical health problems and that are unrelated to a behavioral health diagnosis (NASW, 2016). This billing limitation restricts the ability of health care and community-based organizations to build and sustain interventions that integrate health care and social care to address social needs. Thus, the limitation of social workers' ability to bill for non-mental–health services in a clinical setting by default limits their scope of practice because other sustainable sources of funding for their services often are not available.

One note of caution is warranted here. Laws and regulations governing a profession's scope are generated in political environments and steeped in historical contexts. As such, the current policies governing the scope of practice for health professionals may not reflect the emerging interest in integrating social care into health care delivery, in the effective use of interprofessional teams, and in having all health care workers practicing to the top of their education and training (IOM, 2011). This issue of practicing to the top of one's scope of practice applies to social care workers as well as to traditional health care workers. And emerging workforce professions such as CHWs often have only exclusionary guidance on their scope—there are few states that have statutes or regulations defining their scope of practice, so in most states their work is defined by what other professions claim as exclusive territory (CDC, 2016).

Individual- and organizational-level challenges and barriers affect recruitment and retention efforts and contribute to workforce shortages. For example, in addition to the general reimbursement and scope-of-practice challenges experienced by social workers, individual states differ in their qualifications for licensure, categories of licensure, and scopes of practice. There is no system of license reciprocity or portability among states, making both professional relocation and the provision of telehealth services difficult.

In addition to educating the future health care workforce and training the current workforce about health disparities and the importance of addressing social needs in health care delivery, it is important to make sure that the health care workforce is representative of the demographics of the communities it serves. Substantial variation exists in how well health care and social service occupations reflect the diversity of the U.S. population, with minorities being underrepresented in professions requiring master's level education or higher (HHS, 2017). Employing more underrepresented minority groups in health care may improve how well social care is provided and may better meet the needs of an increasingly diverse U.S. population. Several governmental and nongovernmental bodies have concluded that ensuring that the nation has a diverse health care workforce—especially in terms of gender, cultural, and linguistic representation—is essential (Council on Graduate Medical Education, 2016; HHS, 2006; Wakefield, 2014).

Healthy People 2020 sets goals that include eliminating health disparities, addressing the SDOH, and improving access to high-quality health care (HHS, 2010). Achieving these goals will require the use of culturally informed approaches and the hiring of diverse health care and social services professionals and research investigators who possess the appropriate knowledge and skills. Additional leadership and professional development programs for faculty and students from underrepresented minority groups may help to meet these goals and rectify the underrepresentation of certain demographic groups in the health care workforce. There also is funding for health professions education for minority-serving institutions and underrepresented minorities, including a multitude of programs sponsored by the Health Resources and Services Administration's Bureau of Health Workforce (HRSA, 2018b).

EXAMPLES OF INTERPROFESSIONAL TEAMS THAT ARE ADDRESSING THE FIVE HEALTH CARE SECTOR ACTIVITIES

A range of knowledge, skills, and competencies are necessary to address the five health care sector activities—awareness, adjustment, assistance, alignment, and advocacy. Individual activities require interprofessional approaches, but, more to the point, the range of the activities requires an interprofessional workforce. Highlighted below are several examples of how interprofessional teams around the country are providing social care as a part of health care delivery.

- Hennepin Health in Minnesota is a health care delivery program formed by joint efforts from the Minnesota Department of Human Services, Hennepin County, and the Northpoint Health & Wellness Center.[6] This program seeks to support care delivery reform that can bolster clinical outcomes for patients, both in terms of patient satisfaction and cost. Through multidisciplinary teams, Hennepin Health establishes relationships with patients so its clinicians can best assess the patients' health risk factors and social needs, allowing them to provide the best care coordination possible. The multidisciplinary teams include both clinical and social care workers to ensure that all lifestyle areas that affect health can be covered. These areas include transportation, nutrition, social support, legal, finances, work, and medications.
- Care Neighborhood is a program in Northern California in which CHWs reach out to those most at risk to address their social, medical, and behavioral health care needs in order to reduce costs and decrease the use of hospitals and emergency departments (EDs).[7] Care is delivered by one to two CHWs, who are staff members based at each health center organization and integrated into the medical home team (senior leader champion, social worker, and

[6] For more information, see http://www.healthreform.ct.gov/ohri/lib/ohri/1._hennepin-county-medical-center.pdf (accessed on July 15, 2019).
[7] For more information, see https://www.careinnovations.org/resources/signature-project-care-neighborhood (accessed on July 15, 2019).

nurse). These interdisciplinary teams support the CHWs, whose focus is on member relationship and connection to community resources. The program has been implemented at 8 health center organizations with 12 CHW positions within the Care Neighborhood Network. Once members have been identified by the embedded care team, a clinic-based CHW, with support from a nurse and social worker, assesses and determines next steps. These next steps can include connecting to basic benefits and community resources, connecting to clinic resources and primary care visits, full case management support (navigation, home visits, and care coordination), and integrated behavioral health or housing support services.

- The Bridge model of transitional care is an example of a successful practice-based, cross-disciplinary, and cross-sector care model that addresses social needs (Altfeld et al., 2013; Boutwell et al., 2016; Xiang et al., 2018). Following a hospitalization or rehabilitation stay, Bridge social workers engage with the patient, family members, and inpatient and outpatient providers to ensure smooth discharges that are attentive to social needs and that reinforce primary care engagement. Bridge's protocol applies the social work core competencies of patient engagement, person-in-environment (or systems) theory, resource navigation, and psychotherapeutic techniques. Bridge places significant emphasis on collaboration across the health and social care continuum, sometimes convening all relevant inpatient, primary care, specialty care, community-based, and in-home providers to take part in care continuity calls for particularly complex patients in order to ensure that all the providers understand the patient's care plan and to troubleshoot any issues that arise. In addition to such hospital-driven programs, staff in community-based organizations across the nation who have been trained in Bridge provide transitional care in partnership with hospitals or skilled nursing facilities. In these hospital–community partnerships, the community-based organization generally also provides other services that are commonly included in patients' care plans, such as home-delivered meals or chronic disease self-management classes. The goal is to create a more seamless connection between social care and medical care and thereby to improve health and quality-of-life outcomes for patients and families after an inpatient stay. In various implementation sites with a diverse range of populations, the Bridge model has been found to be associated with increased follow-up with primary care providers, fewer ED visits, and fewer hospital readmissions. Despite these successes, various challenges, including workforce barriers, exist to scaling up and sustaining these cross-sector, interdisciplinary partnerships.

- In an effort to better connect patients with social service agencies that were already available in their area, Geisinger Health System, which operates in parts of Pennsylvania and New Jersey, started a 3-year pilot using community health assistants and social workers to improve resource access.[8] This program was carried out within 5 counties, assisted 16,000 individuals, and closed 24,000 identified "care gaps" in 3 years. The pilot began with five community health assistants and expanded to 36 community health assistants, covering a much wider geography. Community health assistants work with patients to assess their home environment in order to better tailor care access. These health assistants report to a case management team that includes social workers as well as physicians, nurses, and pharmacists. The community health assistants take referrals from primary care physicians and case managers and also directly from community organizations, which can refer someone believed to have a social or health-related need that could benefit from outreach and assistance. In doing so, they make it easier for clinical details to be focused on by case managers.
- When the Massachusetts Department of Public Utilities held a hearing on revising regulations concerning utility shutoffs, attorneys and health care team members from Boston Medical Center were able to successfully advocate for protection for high-risk patients during the winter season.[9] This was achieved through the Boston Medical Center's medical–legal partnership, a combined effort that involves attorneys, nurses, doctors, and other health team members. This partnership was able to offer on-site legal clinics within the medical center and screening that identified high-risk patients (such as those with sickle cell disease and asthma) whose health would suffer from utility power cuts. The screening protocol was then combined with training programs for doctors, to ensure that the correct information for demonstrating medical need was included in protection letters for patients. This combined effort protected 193 people during the first year alone and led to a joint testimony that resulted in the regulation itself being changed.

---

[8] For more information, see https://www.bettercareplaybook.org/_blog/2018/16/geisinger-health-system-deploys-community-health-workers-address-social-determinants (accessed on July 16, 2019).

[9] For more information, see https://medical-legalpartnership.org/response/utilities-case-study (accessed on July 16, 2019).

FINDINGS

- Effectively integrating social care into the delivery of health care requires effective interprofessional teams that include experts in social care.
- The social care workforce can include many types of workers. Social workers are specialists in providing social care who have a long history of working within health care delivery. Models that include community health workers show promise. As models continue to evolve and develop, roles may expand for other workers, such as social service navigators, aides, and assistants; trained volunteers; home health aides and personal care aides; and family caregivers. Other fields are emerging to meet the social needs of older adults (e.g., gerontology) and other specific populations. Integrating other professions—such as lawyers through medical–legal partnerships—also holds promise.
- Understanding the role each member of an interprofessional team plays in the awareness, adjustment, assistance, alignment, and advocacy activities is important for ensuring effective collaboration among team members and for maximizing their ability to address patients' social needs.
- In order to effectively address social care in the delivery of health care, interprofessional team members should operate at their full scope of practice. Federal, state, and institutional barriers limit the scope of practice and the full use of social workers and other social care workers in caring for patients, such as in providing care management as part of an interprofessional team.
- For interprofessional teams to effectively address social care in the context of health care financing structures need to be aligned. Federal, state, and institutional barriers exist that may limit the adequate payment of social workers, gerontologists, and other social care workers.
- Research is needed on workforce issues related to integrating social care and health care, including studying the effect on health and financial outcomes of various configurations of the health care workforce intended to better address the social needs of the population served.

REFERENCES

AACN (American Association of Colleges of Nursing). 2008. *The essentials of baccalaureate education for professional nursing practice.* http://www.aacnnursing.org/portals/42/publications/baccessentials08.pdf (accessed May 26, 2019).

ACGME/ABFM (Accreditation Council for Graduate Medical Education and American Board of Family Medicine). 2015. *The Family Medicine Milestone Project.* https://www.acgme.org/Portals/0/PDFs/Milestones/FamilyMedicineMilestones.pdf (accessed May 26, 2019).

AGHE (Association for Gerontology in Higher Education). 2014. *Gerontology competencies for undergraduate and graduate education.* Washington, DC: Association for Gerontology in Higher Education. https://www.aghe.org/images/aghe/competencies/gerontology_competencies.pdf (accessed May 24, 2019).

AGHE. 2019. *Learn about careers in aging.* Association for Gerontology in Higher Education. https://www.pdx.edu/ioa/sites/www.pdx.edu.ioa/files/learnaboutcareersinaging.pdf (accessed May 24, 2019).

Altfeld, S. J., K. Pavle, W. Rosenberg, and I. Shure. 2013. Integrating care across settings: The Illinois Transitional Care Consortium's Bridge model. *Generations* 36(4):98–101. https://www.apa.org/careers/resources/guides/careers (accessed May 24, 2019).

Ambrose-Miller, W., and R. Ashcroft. 2016. Challenges faced by social workers as members of interprofessional collaborative health care teams. *Health & Social Work* 41(2):101–109.

APHA (American Public Health Association). 2019. *Community health workers.* https://www.apha.org/apha-communities/member-sections/community-health-workers (accessed April 20, 2019).

BLS (Bureau of Labor Statistics). 2019. *What lawyers do.* https://www.bls.gov/ooh/legal/lawyers.htm (accessed March 25, 2019).

Bodenheimer, T., and C. Sinsky. 2014. From triple to quadruple aim: Care of the patient requires care of the provider. *Annals of Family Medicine* 12(6):573–576.

Boutwell, A. E., M. B. Johnson, and R. Watkins. 2016. Analysis of a social work–based model of transitional care to reduce hospital readmissions: Preliminary data. *Journal of the American Geriatrics Society* 64(5):1104–1107.

Bride, B. E. 2007. Prevalence of secondary traumatic stress among social workers. *Social Work* 52(1):63–70.

Buhler-Wilkerson, K. 1993. Bringing care to the people: Lillian Wald's legacy to public health nursing. *American Journal of Public Health* 32(12):1778–1786.

California Department of Health Care Services. 2019. *Home and community-based services (HCBS) billing codes and reimbursement rates.* https://files.medi-cal.ca.gov (accessed August 20, 2019).

Cate, O. T. 2013. Nuts and bolts of entrustable professional activities. *Journal of Graduate Medical Education* 5(1):157–158.

CDC (Centers for Disease Control and Prevention). 2016. *A summary of state community health worker laws.* https://www.cdc.gov/dhdsp/pubs/docs/SLFS-Summary-State-CHW-Laws.pdf (accessed August 13, 2019).

Committee on Training in Primary Care Medicine and Dentistry. 2016. *Addressing the social determinants of health: The role of health professions educations.* https://www.hrsa.gov/advisorycommittees/bhpradvisory/actpcmd/actpcmd_13th_report_sdh_final.pdf (accessed August 20, 2019).

Council on Graduate Medical Education. 2016. *Supporting diversity in the health professions.* https://www.hrsa.gov/advisorycommittees/bhpradvisory/cogme/Publications/diversityresourcepaper.pdf (accessed August 20, 2019).

De Marchis, E., M. Knox, D. Hessler, R. Willard-Grace, J. N. Olayiwola, L. E. Peterson, K. Grumbach, and L. M. Gottlieb. 2019. Physician burnout and higher clinic capacity to address patients' social needs. *Journal of the American Board of Family Medicine* 32(1):69–78.

Doobay-Persaud, A., M. D. Adler, T. R. Bartell, N. E. Sheneman, M. D. Martinez, K. A. Mangold, P. Smith, and K. M. Sheehan. 2019. Teaching the social determinants of health in undergraduate medical education: A scoping review. *Journal of General Internal Medicine* 34(5):720–730.

Eelen, S., S. Bauwens, C. Baillon, W. Distelmans, E. Jacobs, and A. Verzelen. 2014. The prevalence of burnout among oncology professionals: Oncologists are at risk of developing burnout. *Psychooncology* 23(12):1415–1422.

Ellner, A. L., and R. S. Phillips. 2017. The coming primary care revolution. *Journal of General Internal Medicine* 32(4):380–386.

Family Caregiver Alliance. 2016. *Caregiver statistics: Demographics.* https://www.caregiver.org/caregiver-statistics-demographics (accessed March 20, 2019).

Fee, E., and M. E. Garofalo. 2010. Florence Nightingale and the Crimean War. *American Journal of Public Health* 100(9):1591.

Fraser, M. W., B. M. Lombardi, S. Wu, L. de Saxe Zerden, E. L. Richman, and E. P. Fraher. 2018. Integrated primary care and social work: A systematic review. *Journal of the Society for Social Work and Research* 9(2):175–215.

Frenk, J., L. Chen, Z. A. Bhutta, J. Cohen, N. Crisp, T. Evans, H. Fineberg, P. Garcia, Y. Ke, P. Kelley, B. Kistnasamy, A. Meleis, D. Naylor, A. Pablos-Mendez, S. Reddy, S. Scrimshaw, J. Sepulveda, D. Serwadda, and H. Zurayk. 2010. Health professionals for a new century: Transforming education to strengthen health systems in an interdependent world. *The Lancet* 376(9756):1923–1958.

Fulmer, T., L. Guadagno, C. Bitondo, and M. T. Connolly. 2004. Progress in elder abuse screening and assessment instruments. *Journal of the American Geriatrics Society* 52(2):297–304.

Gard, L. A., J. Peterson, C. Miller, N. Ghosh, Q. Youmans, A. Didwania, S. D. Persell, M. Jean-Jacques, P. Ravenna, M. J. O'Brien, and M. S. Goel. 2018. Social determinants of health training in U.S. primary care residency programs: A scoping review. *Academic Medicine* 94(1):135–143.

Garfield, C., and S. Kangovi. 2019. *Integrating community health workers into health care teams without coopting them.* Health Affairs blog. https://www.healthaffairs.org/do/10.1377/hblog20190507.746358/full (accessed August 6, 2019).

Gehlert, S., and T. Browne. 2011. *Handbook of health and social work.* Hoboken, NJ: John Wiley & Sons.

Glaser, B., and E. Suter. 2016. Interprofessional collaboration and integration as experienced by social workers in health care. *Social Work in Health Care* 55(5):395–408.

Greer, P. J., Jr., D. R. Brown, L. G. Brewster, O. G. Lage, K. F. Esposito, E. B. Whisenant, F. W. Anderson, N. K. Castellanos, T. A. Stefano, and J. A. Rock. 2018. Socially accountable medical education: An innovative approach at Florida International University Herbert Wertheim College of Medicine. *Academic Medicine* 93(1):60–65.

Hart, S. M., and A. M. Warren. 2013. Understanding nurses' work: Exploring the links between changing work, labour relations, workload, stress, retention and recruitment. *Economic and Industrial Democracy* 36(2):305–329.

Heisler, E. J. 2018. *The mental health workforce: A primer.* Congressional Research Service. https://fas.org/sgp/crs/misc/R43255.pdf (accessed May 26, 2019).

HHS (U.S. Department of Health and Human Services). 2006. *The rationale for diversity in the health professions: A review of the evidence.* Washington, DC: U.S. Government Printing Office.

HHS. 2010. *HHS announces the nation's new health promotion and disease prevention agenda.* healthypeople.gov/sites/default/files/DefaultPressRelease_1.pdf (accessed August 13, 2019).

HHS. 2017. *Sex, race, and ethnic diversity of U.S. health occupations (2011–2015).* Rockville, MD: U.S. Department of Health and Human Services. https://bhw.hrsa.gov/sites/default/files/bhw/nchwa/diversityushealthoccupations.pdf (accessed May 26, 2019).

Hoge, M. A., J. A. Morris, M. Laraia, A. Pomerantz, and T. Farley. 2014. *Core competencies for integrated behavioral health and primary care.* Washington, DC: SAMHSA-HRSA Center for Integrated Health Solutions.

Houston, R., and R. Mahadevan. 2015. *Supporting social service delivery through Medicaid accountable care organizations: Early state efforts.* Center for Health Care Strategies. https://www.chcs.org/media/Supporting-Social-Service-Delivery-Final_0212151.pdf (accessed May 26, 2019).

HRSA (Health Resources and Services Administration). 2016. *Addressing the social determinants of health: The role of health professions education.* https://www.hrsa.gov/advisorycommittees/bhpradvisory/actpcmd/actpcmd_13th_report_sdh_final.pdf (accessed August 13, 2019).

HRSA 2018a. *Behavioral health workforce projections, 2016–2030.* National Center for Health Workforce Analysis. https://bhw.hrsa.gov/sites/default/files/bhw/health-workforce-analysis/research/projections/Behavioral-Health-Workforce-Projections.pdf (accessed May 26, 2019).

HRSA. 2018b. *Health careers.* https://bhw.hrsa.gov/grants/healthcareers (accessed May 26, 2019).

IOM (Institute of Medicine). 2003a. *Health professions education: A bridge to quality.* Washington, DC: The National Academies Press.

IOM. 2003b. *Unequal treatment: Confronting racial and ethnic disparities in health care.* Washington, DC: The National Academies Press.

IOM. 2008. *Retooling for an aging America: Building the health care workforce.* Washington, DC: The National Academies Press.

IOM. 2011. *The future of nursing: Leading change, advancing health.* Washington, DC: The National Academies Press.

IOM. 2012. *The mental health and substance use workforce for older adults: In whose hands?* Washington, DC: The National Academies Press.

IOM. 2015. *Measuring the impact of interprofessional education on collaborative practice and patient outcomes.* Washington, DC: The National Academies Press.

IPEC (Interprofessional Education Collaborative). 2011. *Core competencies for interprofessional collaborative practice.* https://www.aacom.org/docs/default-source/insideome/ccrpt05-10-11.pdf?sfvrsn=77937f97_2 (accessed May 26, 2019).

Jack, H. E., S. D. Arabadjis, L. Sun, E. E. Sullivan, and R. S. Phillips. 2017. Impact of community health workers on use of healthcare services in the United States: A systematic review. *Journal of General Internal Medicine* 32(3):325–344.

Kangovi, S., N. Mitra, L. Turr, H. Huo, D. Grande, and J. A. Long. 2017. A randomized controlled trial of a community health worker intervention in a population of patients with multiple chronic diseases: Study design and protocol. *Contemporary Clinical Trials* 53:115–121.

Kangovi, S., N. M. Mitra, L. Norton, R. Harte, X. Zhao, T. Carter, D. Grande, and J. A. Long. 2018. Effect of community health worker support on clinical outcomes of low-income patients across primary care facilities: A randomized clinical trial. *JAMA Internal Medicine* 178(12):1635–1643.

Kim, L. Y., D. E. Rose, L. M. Soban, S. E. Stockdale, L. S. Meredith, S. T. Edwards, C. D. Helfrich, and L. V. Rubenstein. 2018. Primary care tasks associated with provider burnout: Findings from a Veterans Health Administration survey. *Journal of General Internal Medicine* 33(1):50–56.

La Motte, E. 2012. The nurse as a social worker. *Public Health Nursing* 29(2):185–187.

Leipzig, R. M., K. Sauvigne, L. J. Granville, G. M. Harper, L. M. Kirk, S. A. Levine, L. Mosqueda, S. M. Parks, H. M. Fernandez, and J. Busby-Whitehead. 2014. What is a geriatrician? American Geriatrics Society and Association of Directors of Geriatric Academic Programs end-of-training entrustable professional activities for geriatric medicine. *Journal of the American Geriatrics Society* 62(5):924–929.

Lin, V. W., J. Lin, and X. Zhang. 2016. U.S. social worker workforce report card: Forecasting nationwide shortages. *Social Work* 61(1):7–15.

Lombardi, B. M., L. de Saxe Zerden, and E. L. Richman. 2017. Toward a better understanding of social workers on integrated care teams. http://www.behavioralhealthworkforce.org/wp-content/uploads/2018/04/Y2FA2P2_UNC-Social-Work-Full-Report.pdf (accessed August 20, 2019).

Long, P., M. Abrams, A. Milstein, G. Anderson, K. Lewis Apton, M. Lund Dahlberg, and D. Whicher (eds.). 2017. *Effective care for high-need patients: Opportunities for improving outcomes, value, and health*. Washington, DC: National Academy of Medicine.

Malcarney, M. B., P. Pittman, L. Quigley, K. Horton, and N. Seiler. 2017. The changing roles of community health workers. *Health Services Research* 52(Suppl 1):360–382.

Mangold, K. A., T. R. Bartell, A. A. Doobay-Persaud, M. D. Adler, and K. M. Sheehan. 2019. Expert consensus on inclusion of the social determinants of health in undergraduate medical education curricula. *Academic Medicine*, January 14 [Epub ahead of print].

Martin, U., and S. P. Schinke. 1998. Organizational and individual factors influencing job satisfaction and burnout of mental health workers. *Journal of Social Work in Health Care* 28(2):51–62.

Martsolf, G. R., D. J. Mason, J. Sloan, C. G. Sullivan, and A. M. Villarruel. 2017. *Nurse-designed care models and culture of health*. Santa Monica, CA: RAND Corporation.

Medves, J., C. Godfrey, C. Turner, M. Paterson, M. Harrison, L. MacKenzie, and P. Durando. 2010. Systematic review of practice guideline dissemination and implementation strategies for healthcare teams and team-based practice. *International Journal of Evidence-Based Healthcare* 8(2):79–89.

Molyneux, J. 2001. Interprofessional teamworking: what makes teams work well? *Journal of interprofessional care* 15(1):29–35.

Mullan, F. 2017. Social mission in health professions education: Beyond Flexner. *JAMA* 318(2):122–123.

NACHW (National Association of Community Health Workers). 2019. *NACHW home page*. https://nachw.org (accessed May 26, 2019).

NASEM (National Academies of Sciences, Engineering, and Medicine). 2016a. *A framework for educating health professionals to address the social determinants of health*. Washington, DC: The National Academies Press.

NASEM. 2016b. *Systems practices for the care of socially at-risk populations*. Washington, DC: The National Academies Press.

NASEM. 2017. *Strengthening the workforce to support community living and participation for older adults and individuals with disabilities*. Washington, DC: The National Academies Press.

NASHP (National Academy for State Health Policy). 2017. *State Community Health Worker Models*. https://nashp.org/state-community-health-worker-models (accessed August 8, 2019).

NASW (National Association of Social Workers). 2005. *NASW standards for clinical social work in social work practice*. https://www.socialworkers.org/LinkClick.aspx?fileticket=YOg4qdefLBE%3D&portalid=0 (accessed August 20, 2019).

NASW. 2016. *NASW standards for social work practice in health care settings*. https://www.socialworkers.org/LinkClick.aspx?fileticket=fFnsRHX-4HE%3D&portalid=0 (accessed May 26, 2019).

NC DHHS (North Carolina Department of Health and Human Services). 2019. *Community health worker initiative*. https://www.ncdhhs.gov/about/department-initiatives/healthy-opportunities/community-health-worker-initiative (accessed April 15, 2019).

Newman, L., F. Baum, S. Javanparast, K. O'Rourke, and L. Carlon. 2015. Addressing social determinants of health inequities through settings: A rapid review. *Health Promotion International* 30:126–143.

Olayiwola, J. N., R. Willard-Grace, K. Dubé, D. Hessler, R. Shunk, K. Grumbach, and L. Gottlieb. 2018. Higher perceived clinic capacity to address patients' social needs associated with lower burnout in primary care providers. *Journal of Health Care for the Poor and Underserved* 29(1):415–429.

Olds, D. L., L. Sadler, and H. Kitzman. 2007. Programs for parents of infants and toddlers: Recent evidence from randomized trials. *Journal of Child Psychology and Psychiatry* 48(3–4):355–391.

Pantell, M. S., E. De Marchis, A. Bueno, and L. M. Gottlieb. 2019. Practice capacity to address patients' social needs and physician satisfaction and perceived quality of care. *Annals of Family Medicine* 17(1):42–45.

Parks, S. M., G. M. Harper, H. Fernandez, K. Sauvigne, and R. M. Leipzig. 2014. American Geriatrics Society/Association of Directors of Geriatric Academic Programs curricular milestones for graduating geriatric fellows. *Journal of the American Geriatric Society* 62(5):930–935.

Pecukonis, E., O. Doyle, S. Acquavita, E. Aparicio, M. Gibbons, and T. Vanidestine. 2013. Interprofessional leadership training in MCH social work. *Social Work Health Care* 52(7):625–641.

Regenstein, M., J. Trott, A. Williamson, and J. Theiss. 2018. Addressing social determinants of health through medical–legal partnerships. *Health Affairs (Millwood)* 37(3):378–385.

Reinhard, S., C. Levine, and S. Samis. 2012. *Home alone: Family caregivers providing complex chronic care*. AARP's Public Policy Institute. https://www.aarp.org/content/dam/aarp/research/public_policy_institute/health/home-alone-family-caregivers-providing-complex-chronic-care-rev-AARP-ppi-health.pdf (accessed May 26, 2019).

Reuben, D. B., L. Levy-Storms, M. N. Yee, M. Lee, K. Cole, M. Waite, L. Nichols, and J. C. Frank. 2004. Disciplinary split: A threat to geriatrics interdisciplinary team training. *Journal of the American Geriatrics Society* 52(6):1000–1006.

Rosenthal, E. L., C. H. Rush, and C. G. Allen. 2016. *Understanding scope and competencies: A contemporary look at the United States community health worker field*. https://www.healthreform.ct.gov/ohri/lib/ohri/work_groups/chw/chw_c3_report.pdf (accessed May 26, 2019).

Siegel, J., D. L. Coleman, and T. James. 2018. Integrating social determinants of health into graduate medical education: A call for action. *Academic Medicine* 93(2):159–162.

Sims, S., G. Hewitt, and R. Harris. 2015. Evidence of collaboration, pooling of resources, learning and role blurring in interprofessional healthcare teams: a realist synthesis. *Journal of Interprofessional Care* 29 (1):20–25.

Tahan, H. A., W. T. Downey, and D. L. Huber. 2006. Case managers' roles and functions: Commission for Case Manager Certification's 2004 research, part II. *Lippincott's Case Manager* 11(2):71–87, quiz 88–89.

USC (University of Southern California). 2019. *Do you know the difference between micro-, mezzo- and macro-level social work?* https://dworakpeck.usc.edu/news/do-you-know-the-difference-between-micro-mezzo-and-macro-level-social-work (accessed May 24, 2019).

Wakefield, M. 2014. Improving the health of the nation: HRSA's mission to achieve health equity. *Public Health Reports* 129(Suppl 2):3–4.

Warshaw, G. A., and E. J. Bragg. 2014. Preparing the health care workforce to care for adults with Alzheimer's disease and related dementias. *Health Affairs (Millwood)* 33(4):633–641.

WHO (World Health Organization). 2010a. *Framework for action on interprofessional education and collaborative practice*. Geneva, Switzerland: World Health Organization. https://www.who.int/hrh/resources/framework_action/en (accessed August 13, 2019).

WHO. 2010b. *Global experience of community health workers for delivery of health related millennium development goals*. Geneva, Switzerland: World Health Organization. https://www.who.int/workforcealliance/knowledge/resources/chwreport/en (accessed August 13, 2019).

Williams, D. R., M. V. Costa, A. O. Odunlami, and S. A. Mohammed. 2008. Moving upstream: How interventions that address the social determinants of health can improve health and reduce disparities. *Journal of Public Health Management & Practice* 14(Suppl):S8–S17.

Xiang, X., A. Zuverink, W. Rosenberg, and E. Mahmoudi. 2018. Social work-based transitional care intervention for super utilizers of medical care: A retrospective analysis of the bridge model for super utilizers. *Social Work in Health Care* 14:1–16.

Zarrella, D. 2005. *Resource manual: Social workers & social work services as defined in Medicare law & regulations*. National Association of Social Works. https://www.socialworkers.org/LinkClick.aspx?fileticket=IyaZ9lqQfLQ%3D&portalid=0 (accessed May 26, 2019).

Zomorodi, M., T. Odom, N. C. Askew, C. R. Leonard, K. A. Sanders, and D. Thompson. 2018. Hotspotting: Development of an interprofessional education and service learning program for care management in home care patients. *Nurse Educator* 43(5):247–250.

4

Leveraging Data and Digital Tools

Integrating social care into health care—through awareness, adjustment, assistance, alignment, and advocacy—requires the coordination of information, people, and services across and between organizations and across sectors, often in the presence of well-established silos. The data from these sectors and services necessary for effective integration are similarly siloed, if they are present at all. To date, successful alignment of services that address social needs and traditional medical care has largely been achieved through human capital–intensive approaches to information sharing, involving unstructured and non-automated information exchanges (e.g., many hours spent on communication via telephone, fax, and email) and marked by a lack of consistency or standardization of data within and between health and social care domains (Onie et al., 2018). Where electronic information is available, the information technology systems are marked by a general absence of interoperability and by unequal investments in information management infrastructure for different types of providers (NCCBH, 2012). However, relying on manual approaches to coordinate information in the support of integrated care is costly, inefficient, and difficult to scale, thus limiting the seamless implementation of near-upstream approaches to addressing social needs.

By leveraging data and technology, the health care sector and its social care partners have an opportunity to improve the efficiency, effectiveness, and sustainability of efforts that address health-related social needs as a regular component of health care delivery (Dameff et al., 2019). In this chapter, the committee has identified critical opportunities that must be addressed in order to create an environment in which data and digital tools have the potential to meaningfully affect social care integration into health care, leading to a more effective and efficient set of care models. These opportunities also stand to improve the experience for the people served and the workforce serving them.

LAYING THE FOUNDATION FOR DATA AND TECHNOLOGY TO DRIVE SOCIAL CARE INTEGRATION IN HEALTH CARE

The past decade has seen a dramatic technological transformation within the health care sector, driven by large-scale federal policy and, more recently, by new payment models in both the public and private sectors that incentivize major investments in building core information infrastructure in order to better manage patient populations. The federal government has played a substantial role in steering and financing the digitization of the health care experience for Americans. The Health Information Technology for Economic and Clinical Health (HITECH) Act of 2009[1] stimulated unprecedented growth in the adoption of electronic health records (EHRs) through a combination of policies, programs, incentives, and penalties. "As of 2017, nearly 9 in 10 (86 percent) of office-based physicians had adopted any EHR, and nearly 4 in 5 (80%) had adopted a certified EHR. Since 2008, office-based physician adoption of any EHRs has more than doubled, from 42% to 86%" (ONC, 2019). The wide adoption of EHRs and electronic information as a more ubiquitous component of many aspects of health care delivery and operations now presents opportunities to harness the power of big data to continuously improve care quality, efficiency, and health outcomes (IOM, 2013).

Federal policy driven by Congress and the U.S. Department of Health and Human Services (HHS) has created a supportive environment for the improved use of data and technology to optimize the health care experience, with a focus on promoting interoperability between disparate systems and providing consumers electronic access to their health and other information. The Centers for Medicare & Medicaid Services (CMS) has provided financial support for and required the use of certified EHR technology by eligible professionals and hospitals under the Medicare and Medicaid EHR Incentive and Promoting Interoperability programs (CMS, 2019c). CMS efforts are coupled with policy efforts by The Office of the National Coordinator for Health Information Technology (ONC), which oversees health information technology (IT) certification and has recently shifted from a focus on driving EHR adoption to

[1] Health Information Technology for Economic and Clinical Health Act. Public Law 111-5, § 13001, 111th Cong. (February 12, 2009).

encouraging the availability of clinical data for providers, payers, and patients (Washington et al., 2017) .

ONC was tasked by the 21st Century Cures Act of 2016[2] to develop a trusted exchange framework to significantly improve data sharing and to administer penalties to any entity engaged in data-blocking practices, such as vendors requesting excessive fees to access health data (Rucker, 2018). This legislation also codified the use of open application program interface (API) technology to connect third-party apps to health IT systems in the same way many popular commercial applications use APIs to connect and share data across disparate apps (e.g., Google Maps and Uber). In the spring of 2019, ONC and CMS released notices of proposed rulemaking to advance interoperability, as directed by the 21st Century Cures Act; if finalized as proposed, insurers that offer qualified health plans through and outside of the federal marketplace, Medicare Advantage plans, Medicaid- and Children's Health Insurance Program (CHIP)-managed care organizations, and state Medicaid and CHIP agencies that offer fee-for-service programs would be required to implement an open API to allow third-party app access to claims data when such access has been approved by the patient (CMS, 2019b).

HHS is not the only agency with health data under its purview; the Federal Health Architecture (FHA), which is transitioning to the Federal Health IT Coordinating Committee, supports interagency collaboration at the federal level and coordinates among more than 20 federal agencies to enhance health information exchange and coordinate services (ONC, 2018). For example, the Blue Button initiative started in 2010 as an effort by the U.S. Department of Veterans Affairs (VA) to give veterans more ready access to their medical records; HHS expanded upon the standards developed by the VA to give patients view, download, and transmit access to their health data in a standard format (ONC, 2014). CMS is now advancing Blue Button 2.0, an initiative that uses standards-based API technology to enable patients to share their medical data with trusted apps and programs (CMS, 2019a).

Federal policies to advance interoperable health data systems have been joined by innovation in the private sector, including the exponentially growing capacity of cloud-based data storage and associated big data analytic opportunities. The past decade has seen a dramatic evolution of computing and analytic technologies, which promises to unveil new insights and interventions previously unavailable with traditional research methods and data availability (Raghupathi and Raghupathi, 2014). Artificial intelligence and machine-learning techniques have substantial potential to transform the use of health care data by enabling much more

[2] 21st Century Cures Act. Public Law 114-255, 114th Cong. (December 13, 2016).

sophisticated analytics to drive targeted interventions and improve efficiency (Beam and Kohane, 2018).

The private sector has been an important partner in federal efforts to improve data availability for individual-level care and population health. Such efforts as the High Level 7 (HL7) Argonaut Project[3] and the CARIN Alliance[4] are advancing data standards and technological capabilities and working to develop a "trust framework" that allows consumers' data to be in machine-readable format and able to be aggregated by a trusted app or other third party (Dameff et al., 2019). The regulatory framework that HHS has proposed would promote greater use of third parties such as health information exchange organizations that can aggregate data across disparate systems to create longitudinal health records and that could also incorporate social care data. Venture capital firms have also invested heavily in health technology—with nearly $8.1 billion invested in digital health startups in 2018 alone—and have evinced a growing interest in platforms that support integrated care for patient populations with unmet social needs (Day and Zweig, 2018). As one example, Town Hall Ventures seeks to partner with mission-driven entrepreneurs and targets its investments in "businesses that serve underserved populations … [including] a range of opportunities across health care technology and services, as well as areas which address social determinants of health" (Town Hall Ventures, 2019). It remains to be seen whether using private capital in the social care arena will result in equitable improvements in access, or instead aggravate existing disparities in the health and social care systems.

This creation of a digitized health care system is associated with a growing set of opportunities to leverage data and digital tools that can not only improve health care, but also support efforts aimed at identifying social risks and addressing social needs along the spectrum described in Chapter 2. As other sectors, particularly those involved with the consumer experience (e.g., retail, banking, and entertainment), have become digitized, there has become a largely untapped opportunity to better incorporate data from multiple sources beyond the EHR to establish a broader view of the health status of individuals and communities, inclusive of health-related social factors. For example, eligibility and enrollment files for social services programs and experiences with care and services all may contribute to creating a more complete picture of individuals' health needs and drivers. In addition, there is a flurry of activity aimed at using other data, including community-level information such as hardship indices or information on the availability of healthy food or public transportation. Other efforts are using personal and community

[3] HL7 International (2019).

[4] CARIN Alliance (2019).

retail patterns (Messer et al., 2006). Researchers and businesses are exploring the potential of using patient- and neighborhood-level social need data to inform risk models and predict the need for wrap-around interventions or referrals to social services (Kasthurirathne et al., 2018).

The value of advanced analytic approaches in driving effective resource deployment and service delivery will depend on the quality and comprehensiveness of the available data. As an example, health care claims and encounter data, which are often used to risk-stratify patients for population health interventions, have limited utility in predicting hospital readmissions for individuals with social risk factors like homelessness or social isolation because information about social risk factors is more likely to be found in clinical notes (Navathe et al., 2018). Administrative data have even less value in identifying the need for or use of social care services for most people with social needs. Thus, efforts to enrich core datasets to include sociodemographics, family caregiver status, social interactions, consumer habits, and even social media use will be key to unlocking the potential of analytic tools and care models (Beam and Kohane, 2018).

Beyond the data and their application are new digital tools that are only just beginning to be used to address social risks and social needs. Smartphones, mobile technology, and the Internet are becoming more available even in low-income communities, and patients and their caregivers are increasingly accustomed to accessing information and services through a digital layer (Pew Research Center, 2019). The ease of use, autonomy, and flexibility that technology provides has transformed virtually every domain of modern life—from the way that most people shop to the way they maintain connections with friends and family. One notable exception to this is in accessing and coordinating health care and social care services. Yet, it is precisely in this space where the potential of technology to meaningfully enhance the provider and consumer experience is so great. Technology can help reduce the cognitive burden that individuals experience when having to navigate complex, disconnected systems to access health care and social care services by streamlining consent processes and information sharing (Shah et al., 2018). Unfortunately, much of the promise of big data and analytics for integrating social care with health care remains unrealized (NAAAA, 2015).

THE EVOLVING ROLE OF DATA AND TECHNOLOGY IN ENHANCING SOCIAL CARE AND ITS INTEGRATION IN HEALTH CARE

In Chapter 2 the committee identified five complementary types of activities that health care systems can adopt to strengthen social care integration—awareness, adjustment, assistance, alignment, and advocacy.

Data and technology are already being leveraged in each of these areas and will have an increasingly important role to play across the spectrum of integration. In this section the committee provides examples of data sources and technology applications that may improve the effectiveness and efficiency of field efforts to address the social determinants of health (SDOH) in the health care environment. These uses of data and digital tools also stand to improve the ability to systematically evaluate care and financing models and build a stronger evidence base to support integration (see Table 4-1). The digital systems for the social care environment should be developed building on lessons learned from federal efforts to digitize the health care system (Reisman, 2017). These lessons include from the outset requiring non-proprietary standards to enable

TABLE 4-1
Potential Sources of Data and Digital Tools to Support the Integration of Social Care into Health Care

Social Care Integration Spectrum	Potential Data Sources			
	Health care claims	Structured and unstructured data from electronic health record	Social determinants data from surveys	Retail and purchasing data
Awareness	X	X	X	X
Adjustment	X	X	X	X
Assistance	X	X	X	X
Alignment	X	X	X	X
Advocacy	X	X	X	X

Social Care Integration Spectrum	Potential Applied Analytic and Technology Tools			
	Predictive analytics	Natural-language processing of unstructured data	Geocoding/hotspotting	Point-of-care decision support
Awareness	X	X	X	
Adjustment	X	X		X
Assistance	X	X	X	X
Alignment		X	X	
Advocacy	X	X	X	X

interoperability and setting expectations of data sharing as a condition of participation in the health ecosystem. The digital systems should also be developed with input from persons with expertise in social care.

Awareness

Data and digital tools are instrumental to increasing the health care sector's awareness of social risks. The tools and processes needed to facilitate the systematic assessment of individual-level, health-related social needs is an area of active development. A better understanding of a person's social context is integral to identifying the presence of risk factors, such as food insecurity or exposure to violence that can have a substantial

	Community-level information (e.g., census)	Evidence-based protocols for decision support	Eligibility criteria for social services programs	Health and social program enrollment options	Local social determinants of health findings	Local public policy and statutes
	X					
	X	X				
	X	X	X	X		
	X	X	X	X	X	X
	X	X	X	X	X	X

	Augmented intelligence	Internet of Things	Telehealth and other virtual care	Automated interactions (chat bots, holograms)	Drones and self-driving cars	Digital platforms for interoperability
	X			X		
	X	X	X			
	X	X	X	X	X	
	X	X	X	X		X
	X					

effect on the efficacy of care plans and health outcomes (Billioux et al., 2017). The identification of social factors that relate to health risk is an essential first step toward fulfilling unmet social needs and improving health by connecting people with the social care services. Such needs may occur at the patient level or at the neighborhood and community level, and thus efforts to collect both types of data may help increase awareness. The strengths and limitations of each approach are summarized in Table 4-2.

Most approaches to increasing the awareness of social risks within the health care sector have relied on patient-level data collected through surveys administered during the course of patients' engagement with the health system (Freij et al., 2018; Gottlieb et al., 2018) (see Chapter 2 for examples; also see Box 4-1). Such approaches are endorsed by professional and medical organizations in the United States, but they have not been widely implemented or formally evaluated (AAFP, 2019a; Daniel et al., 2018).

The health care sector has been active in testing and learning the best approaches for deploying technology to identify social risk, though there is not yet a best practice or standard. While substantial progress has been made in better assessing social and environmental risk factors as a means of predicting and improving health outcomes, there remain many challenges with screening mechanisms and the utility and reliability of the data they produce (Byhoff et al., 2018; Gottlieb et al., 2018). As noted in Chapter 2, when individuals interact with the health care system, it presents an opportunity to screen them for social risk information, but there are few standard instruments and minimal research to support the validity of such screening tools.

Part of building screening capabilities into the clinical workflow includes the integration of data on health-related social risks into the EHR, which already houses important medical information. Federally qualified health centers (FQHCs) have been early adopters of tools to assess the social risk of the underserved patient populations served by these organizations; the Protocol for Responding to and Assessing Patients' Assets, Risks, and Experiences (PRAPARE) assessment tool developed by the National Association of Community Health Centers (see Box 4-1) helps FQHCs better coordinate clinical and non-clinical care by collecting and documenting social risk data in the EHR (NACHC et al., 2016).

Currently, no uniform, accepted data model exists for representing social determinants in an EHR (Cantor and Thorpe, 2018). Therefore, while the benefits to EHR integration are numerous, the investment required to successfully achieve functional integration can be substantial (Gold et al., 2018) (also see Chapter 6). A standard for non-medical data is integral to translation of social determinants information into meaningful

TABLE 4-2
Strengths and Limitations of Patient- and Neighborhood-Level Social Determinants of Health Data Application

Health Data	Patient-Level Interventions	Neighborhood-Level Interventions
Patient-level data	*Strengths:* Screening data collected directly from patients are likely more sensitive and specific to condition. Screening and intervention are both in context of shared clinical decision making, so can more closely tie interventions to patients' priority needs.	*Strengths:* Using a patient lens may increase the health care system's engagement in upstream activities. Data may be more quickly accessible and aggregated.
	Limitations: Cost of screening entire clinical population. Sampling bias and social desirability bias may affect patients' responses to health care practitioners. High cost of intervening at individual level to address neighborhood-level issues (e.g., housing inadequacy, food deserts).	*Limitations:* Sampling bias and social desirability bias may affect patients' responses to health care practitioners. Subject to "exception fallacy": Patients from health care system may not reflect neighborhood population adequately.
Neighborhood-level data	*Strengths:* Increases health care system's engagement in upstream, neighborhood-level activities. Potential to focus on entire population facing health consequences, which could enhance value of interventions.	*Strengths:* Uses a population-level lens; may be more "objective." More capacity to affect population-level change.
	Limitations: Subject to "ecological fallacy": Some patients in this neighborhood may not be at higher risk. Lack of timely and detailed data limits depth of understanding. Potential to increase stigma. Potential to reinforce inequity across factors other than neighborhood (i.e., easier to intervene on behalf of relatively healthier individuals in the same neighborhood).	*Limitations:* Can use only social determinants of health data that are available (practitioner has less control over how data are collected). May not have a direct impact on health system's catchment population. Lack of timely data limits ability to monitor and adjust interventions.

SOURCE: Gottlieb et al., 2018. Reprinted with permission from *The Permanente Journal.*

Box 4-1 **Awareness Approach: PRAPARE Tool for Federally Qualified Health Centers**

"The Protocol for Responding to and Assessing Patients' Assets, Risks, and Experiences (PRAPARE) is a national effort to help health centers and other providers collect the data needed to better understand and act on their patients' social determinants of health" (NACHC, 2019). The PRAPARE assessment tool consists of a set of national core measures as well as a set of optional measures for community priorities. It was informed by research, the experience of existing social risk assessments, and stakeholder engagement. It aligns with national initiatives prioritizing social determinants (e.g., *Healthy People 2020*), measures proposed under the next stage of Meaningful Use, clinical coding under ICD-10, and health centers' Uniform Data System. PRAPARE emphasizes measures that are actionable. PRAPARE electronic health record templates exist for eClinicalWorks, Epic, GE Centricity, and NextGen.

SOURCE: NACHC, 2019.

outcomes or conditions (akin to ICD-10 codes for medical diagnoses) that lend themselves to clinical response; yet, many codes exist that describe social determinants with different coding vocabularies (Arons et al., 2018). Efforts are under way to develop documentation standards and to better align coding vocabularies used in EHRs in order to improve interoperability in this area (IOM, 2014). One such effort is the Gravity Project, led by the Social Interventions Research and Evaluation Network (SIREN), with funding from the Robert Wood Johnson Foundation, which is aimed at developing consensus-based code recommendations for capturing data on food security, housing stability and quality, and transportation access and to ultimately inform an HL7 Fast Healthcare Interoperability Resource implementation guide for priority-use cases (SIREN, 2019).

Ideally, integration of standardized data into EHRs will enable such functionalities as automatic referral to community-based organizations; however, this type of integration with entities outside the health care system will require an increased capacity of community-based organizations to comply with privacy and security standards related to the sharing of protected health information (PHI) as well as the health care sector's willingness to share data. The Office for Civil Rights (OCR) governs the Health Insurance Portability and Accountability Act (HIPAA) and recently solicited public comments in a request for information on provisions of the privacy and security regulations that may impede transformation to a value-based health care system. The request for information noted that some HIPAA-covered entities have been reluctant to share PHI for care coordination purposes for fear of violating HIPAA, even though the rules currently permit disclosure to third parties such as social service agencies or community-based support programs for the purpose of coordinating care and related services (HHS, 2018). OCR also solicited recommendations for improved HIPAA training for covered entities, which could address the knowledge gap in what data-sharing activities are currently permissible.

Organizations also are using big data from a wide range of sources and sectors to paint a detailed picture of social risks and needs at the population level in order to inform place-based community improvement strategies as well as individual interventions. Various tools are in use to integrate neighborhood-level data into EHRs to help inform patient-level interventions. Geographic information system (GIS) tools such as HealthLandscape (AAFP, 2019b) and Texas A&M University's GeoServices (TAMU, 2019) allow for the analysis of geocoded patient datasets (Robert Grahm Center, 2019). These social risk assessment approaches may, for example, help alleviate the burden of primary screening and enhance population-level interventions within the public and private sectors targeted to the zip code level (Auger et al., 2017). They also can be used to track institutional progress on addressing disparities among target communities (Abu-Saad et al., 2018; Cookson et al., 2018; Hanak, 2018). In the case of the Flint water crisis, GIS tools were used to improve the validity of a blood lead level study by analyzing patient data from the precise neighborhoods that had been switched to tap water supplied from a more corrosive source (Hanna-Attisha et al., 2016).

The more common approaches of individual-level data collection for population health surveillance are time and resource-intensive, typically involving either a prolonged face-to-face interaction between the surveyor and the patient or the self-completion of paper surveys directly by patients, with the surveys manually entered and recorded into a database (Richards et al., 2017). The trade-offs between these two approaches of individual-level data collection largely involve compromising either efficiency, in the former case, or the quality and precision of the data gathered in the latter. For example, completing such surveys may add time to the clinical encounter and detract from the time that patients have available to interact with the care team (NASDOH, 2019). There are other challenges as well, including the burden on the patients who are asked to repeatedly describe their social needs, which in some cases may cause them embarrassment or a loss of dignity.

Adjustment

Understanding social risk and social need is only the beginning of addressing those issues. Health systems are deploying data and technology strategies to support the development of individualized care plans and inform clinical care decision making. An immediate benefit derived from assessing social risk is the adjustment of clinical care plans to accommodate for social needs. In making such adjustments, doctors and other clinicians need patients' social risk information to inform their diagnostic and care plan. As an example, people who are homeless may have their diabetic therapeutic regimens hampered by the addition of insulin because they do not have an easy opportunity to store insulin. When transportation poses a barrier to accessing care, a clinician may choose to call a patient to follow up on results of laboratory or diagnostic tests rather than expecting the patient to present for an in-person follow up visit. In addition to using patient-level data to inform patient-level interventions, neighborhood-level data also may help tailor care to maximize the chance of success (see Box 4-2).

Assistance

The health care system is deploying a range of data and technological interventions to assist patients in connecting with resources to address social needs. One evolving area with substantial potential for influence is the development of new technologies to mediate virtual interactions

Box 4-2 Adjustment Approach: Neighborhood-Level Data Inform Patient-Level Interventions

"As part of Cincinnati Children's Hospital Medical Center's commitment to decreasing health inequities, the hospital has selected two local neighborhoods in which to focus disparity-reducing activities. Neighborhoods were chosen on the basis of census and other area-level data showing disproportionately high rates of both all-cause morbidity and underlying risks related to poverty, such as housing instability and poor transportation access (neighborhood level data). Each morning, a multidisciplinary team of physicians, nurses, social workers, and community engagement consultants receives an alert from the electronic health record identifying any child hospitalized from these high-risk neighborhoods. This prompts in-depth chart review and a bedside huddle focused on the potential preventability of the hospitalization, identifiable care gaps (for example, need for vaccinations, overdue for primary care follow-up), and transition needs. When appropriate, patients are connected with additional supports during the hospitalization (for example, social work consultation, connection to a community health worker) and/or specialized transition-related service delivery, such as post discharge nurse home visits, medication delivery, or school-based outreach programs (patient-level intervention)."

SOURCE: Gottlieb et al., 2018.

between individuals and care teams, as well as to deliver goods and services (National Interoperability Collaborative, 2019). When applied to health and social care, these technologies hold the potential to improve access, reduce transaction costs, and enhance engagement. In some clinical environments, this includes the use of tools that have digitized resource guides that make the information searchable and allow for the identification of resources that match patient characteristics such as location, language, or access on public transportation (Alley et al., 2016). Digital resource guides available on the market include those that are produced with community input on available resources and increasingly allow for individuals to "rate" services provided by the social care organizations.

As the health sector transitions to more value-based payment arrangements that hold providers accountable for patient outcomes and the total cost of care, providers and payers have greater incentive to assist patients in addressing unmet social needs. The health sector must decide whether to build capacity to directly assist patients' non-medical needs or, alternatively, to partner with community-based organizations that have experience in addressing social needs and the necessary capacity to address those needs. In the latter scenario, the health sector will also need to consider what data systems can be used in partnering with social care providers. North Carolina, through a public–private partnership, is establishing a shared utility for plans and providers to use across all populations and payers, including Medicare, Medicaid, and commercially insured and uninsured populations, to assist in making referrals to social service providers; one purpose is to avoid the need for each plan and provider to establish a separate referral platform. The referral platform will have a digitized resource directory and a feedback regulated referral functionality to track the outcome of the referrals and collect data on the delivery of social care. As North Carolina transitions to Medicaid managed care in the latter part of 2019, the North Carolina Medicaid program will use this shared utility for the state's Medicaid plans and providers. The state's technology-facilitated assistance platform, NCCARE360, is described in Box 4-3.

Alignment

The committee defined alignment activities as those generally led by health care organizations working to organize social care providers and services in their area. The ultimate goal is to harmonize activity, services, and funding for these resources in order to maximize effectiveness. An example of an organization involved in such an alignment approach—the Route 66 Consortium—is presented in Box 4-4. Because these alignment efforts extend beyond the support of individuals, community-level data

Box 4-3 Assistance Approach: NCCARE360

"NCCARE360 is the first statewide coordinated care network to electronically connect people with identified needs to community resources and allow for a feedback loop on the outcome of that connection." "NCCARE360 is the result of a public-private partnership between NC Department of Health and Human Services and the Foundation for Health Leadership & Innovation." "Through NCCARE360, community partners will have access to:

- A robust statewide resource directory that will include a call center with dedicated navigators, a data team verifying resources and text and chat capabilities.
- A data repository to integrate resource directories across the state to share resource data.
- A shared technology platform that enables health care and human service providers to send and receive secure electronic referrals, seamlessly communicate in real-time, securely share client information and track outcomes.
- A community engagement team working with community-based organizations, social service agencies, health systems, independent providers and more to create a statewide coordinated care network."

"This solution ensures accountability around services delivered, provides a 'no wrong door' approach and closes the loop on every referral made. NCCARE360 implementation started in January 2019. NCCARE360 will be available in every county in North Carolina with full statewide implementation by end of 2020."

SOURCE: NC DHHS, 2019.

including asset maps of local social services and geocoded data population health needs are needed to connect people with social needs with the appropriate resources. Such work will require the sharing of health and social care information across a wide array of community partners and with the consumer. In addition to the use of digital-sharing platforms, the work will benefit from the regular updating of resource guides to keep them current, with care providers' contact information, eligibility criteria, and online enrollment platforms. Social service resource lists that are integrated into the EHR and platforms that support closed-loop referrals (where only the specialist and primary care provider are involved) can support successful care coordination when individuals face care hand-offs between health care and social care providers. Alignment models will also benefit from shared data repositories that can be accessed by all partners to inform the development of resources to fill gaps or reduce redundancy in services identified in asset mapping.

Box 4-4 Alignment Approach: The Route 66 Consortium

"Accountable Health Communities is a partnership between the Centers for Medicare and Medicaid Services and MyHealth Access Network to study if identifying and addressing health-related social needs impacts health care cost and reduces health care utilization. Accountable Health Communities is looking at how factors outside the clinical setting impact the health of patients.

Accountable Health Communities aims to:

- Conduct systematic health-related social needs screenings of patients in partner clinics
- Refer patients to community services that may be able to address the identified social needs
- Navigate Medicare and Medicaid beneficiaries to community service providers in their communities
- Align community partners to optimize capacity to address health-related social needs.

MyHealth is using a mobile screening process that sends a text message with a link to a screening that will identify health-related social needs and provide the patient a list of customized resources to help address the identified needs. This process provides a valuable service to the patient with no additional workload for the healthcare facility.

Accountable Health Communities will focus on the following core areas:

- Housing instability and quality
- Food insecurity
- Utility needs
- Interpersonal violence
- Transportation needs beyond medical transportation.

The study will also provide navigation services for high-risk Medicare and Medicaid patients through the Tulsa and Oklahoma City County Health Departments. The patient will be contacted by a Navigator who will help connect them with community service providers in their area to meet their identified social needs. They will provide follow up support for up to a year."

SOURCE: MyHealth Access Network, 2019.

Advocacy

The committee defined advocacy activities as those in which health care–related organizations work with partner social care agencies to create, develop, or redeploy assets or resources to address health and social care needs. Such changes involve systems-level changes that can affect the community as a whole and therefore require data and digital tools that transcend individual-level information and provide population-level asset and geographic data to enhance alignment models. Advocacy efforts will be best supported by data from inventories of existing local and national best practices of legal and policy frameworks to inform opportunities for change such as in housing policy or transportation (CDC, 2019). These efforts will need to include data resources that are in community-based organizations and governmental organizations that are not typically sharing data with health care, such as departments of urban planning, environment, public works, education, and transportation. The work of the Louisville AIR project and how it addressed asthma with technology, crowdsourcing, cross-sector collaboration, and policy is one such example (see Box 4-5).

CHALLENGES

The committee identified a number of challenges that health care and social care systems are facing in working to use data and technology as part of their efforts to integrate care and services across the continuum, which have been discussed throughout this chapter. None of these challenges is insurmountable, but overcoming them will require deliberate action by policy makers and the private sector. Some will likely also require considerable financial investment. Some of the key challenges are:

- **Access to sufficient social services data and digital infrastructure.** HITECH provided billions of dollars to support the

Box 4-5 Advocacy Approach: AIR Louisville

"Cross-sector partnerships benefit public health by leveraging ideas, resources, and expertise from a wide range of partners. In this study, we documented the process and impact of AIR Louisville (a collaboration forged among the Louisville Metro Government, a nonprofit institute, and a technology company) in successfully tackling a complex public health challenge: asthma. We enrolled residents of Louisville, Kentucky, with asthma and used electronic inhaler sensors to monitor where and when they used medication. We found that the use of the digital health platform achieved positive clinical outcomes, including a 78 percent reduction in rescue inhaler use and a 48 percent improvement in symptom-free days. Moreover, the crowdsourced real-world data on inhaler use, combined with environmental data, led to policy recommendations including enhancing tree canopy, tree removal mitigation, zoning for air pollution emission buffers, recommended truck routes, and developing a community asthma notification system. AIR Louisville represents a model that can be replicated to address many public health challenges by simultaneously guiding individual, clinical, and policy decisions."

SOURCE: Barrett et al., 2018.

transformational digitization of the U.S. health care sector, thus rapidly accelerating the uptake of digital technology by health care providers. The social services sector did not benefit from these funds, and in most cases the IT infrastructure of community-based organizations that provide services is incapable of meeting the data standards, cybersecurity, and other technological needs to build a robust health care and social care data sharing infrastructure (Amarasingham et al., 2018).

- **Lack of data standards for social determinants of health.** "Vendors that are developing products to facilitate the collection and use of social determinants of health data are seeking solutions to data standardization and interoperability challenges" (Freij et al., 2018, p. 2).
- **Interoperability.** The interoperability of health care data continues to improve year over year in the United States, but it still does not meet expectations. This is due largely to business decisions that cause the health care sector to block data. However, efforts to create business incentives for data sharing at the federal level in concert with private-sector action is showing progress (AHA, 2019). The interoperability landscape is already working to build a trust framework and set of incentives for sharing data between health and social care systems. As such, going forward the health care and social sectors will need to agree upon a shared trust framework for data exchange, sharing, and use. Part of building a transparent trust framework will be the need to have meaningful informed consent for individuals (California Governor's Office of Planning and Research, 2018; Illinois Department of Human Services, 2013).
- **Privacy and security.** The data used in some models of social care information will move between health care systems and social services partners who are unaccustomed to the regulatory expectations included in HIPAA that govern the protection of personally identifiable data (see Figure 4-1). All of the organizations involved in this data sharing will need technical assistance to build informed consent for individuals and data sharing arrangements that can support information flow. In addition, some of the data that will be shared or included in risk prediction models will fall outside of HIPAA protections and therefore may require additional regulatory or statutory action (IOM, 2009).
- **Data and technology skills for workforce and patients.** As has been the case with the digitization of other human capital intensive industries, technology can enable skilled workers to focus on more technically complex activities while expanding access and

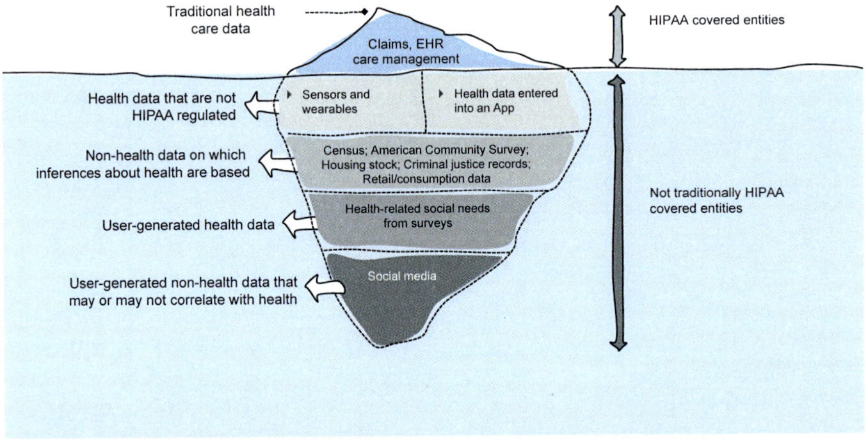

FIGURE 4-1 Protection of data used in health and social care integration.
NOTE: HIPPA = Health Insurance Portability and Accountability Act.
SOURCE: Adapted from Price and Cohen, 2019. Reprinted with permission from *Nature Medicine*.

enhancing operational efficiency. But, to achieve that goal, the health care and social care incumbent and emerging workforce will need to be comfortable with data and technology. Though people working in the health care sector have become more accustomed to and comfortable with data and technology (as a result of the increased utilization of EHRs), the social care sector lags behind in these capabilities and will require adequate training and peer champions to ease the transition (Wyman and SeaChange Capital Partners, 2017).

- **Consumer demand and expectations.** Amid the excitement on the payer and provider side concerning digital technology and its potential to improve the efficiency of resource deployment and overall health outcomes, there has been very little investigation of consumer desires and expectations. It remains to be seen whether and how individual patients (consumers) will embrace the use of data and technology to integrate services in some of the most personal, intimate parts of their lives. As an example, some individuals may not want their physician to know whether they receive meals from a food pantry or how often they sleep in a shelter. Others might be very uncomfortable to know that their health plan is gathering data on their credit score and grocery purchases to determine what type of care management services to offer them.

- **Balancing technology and human capital investments.** Data and technology stand to accelerate the care models that can address and, where needed, mitigate the social factors that influence health. But data and technology alone are not the solution. Absent humanity, those truly with need will not be helped. Technology cannot and should not be a replacement for trusted human relationships. The goal should be to augment human capital and processes rather than supplant them.
- **Inequitable access to technology and unintended consequences.** There are instances when digitizing the social and health care infrastructure can result in negative consequences and exacerbate disparities. Such is the case where states have implemented Medicaid work requirements and required beneficiaries to report work hours online. In Arkansas, which has seen Medicaid coverage losses because of conditioning eligibility on work requirements (Rudowitz et al., 2019), more than half (53 percent) of nonexempt Medicaid beneficiaries that are working the required number of hours still face difficulty complying with the reporting requirement because they are in households with no broadband Internet access (Gangopadhyaya et al., 2018).
- **Ethics of social risk profiling.** Finally, potentially serious ethical considerations will need to be addressed in the application of artificial intelligence and other modalities in decision making and resource allocation for integrating social care into health care (Char et al., 2018; Gottlieb and Alderwick, 2019). Of particular concern is the risk that these technologies replicate or exacerbate the biases within the current social and health care systems that result in disparities in outcomes on the basis of race and ethnicity, sexual orientation, gender identity, history of trauma, or other status.

FINDINGS

- Data and technology have transformed the consumer experience in many sectors of life and are doing so in health care. This is only the beginning of a journey that has unlimited potential to use data and technology to improve effectiveness and transform the consumer experience.
- Billions of dollars in federal resources spurred the digitization of health care through the widespread adoption of the electronic health records and interoperability. Social care has not benefited from the same resources and policy attention as has the health care sector, and it lags far behind in digitization.

- Private equity has supported the health technology economy. Venture capitalists are increasingly investing in health technology startup companies that are working to address the social determinants of health.
- Local efforts to share health care and social care data exist, including an emerging set of private-sector solutions. These are not supported by a strategic national vision, nor coupled with resources or defined technology standards.
- Interoperability and data sharing between health care and social care are hampered by the lack of infrastructure, data standards, and modern technology architecture shared between and among organizations.
- With an increasing number of stakeholders sharing protected health information in order to coordinate care, data privacy and security remain challenging elements to manage. Concerns about compliance with regulations such as those governing health care data (e.g., Health Insurance Portability and Accountability Act information) and social data (e.g., educational information) are barriers to sharing at the local level.
- The deployment of digital approaches to integrating social care into health care may increase existing health disparities by exacerbating the digital divide or codifying bias within health and social systems.
- There is a paucity of rigorous research that can inform a collective understanding of best practices and outcomes of efforts to integrate social care with health care. Access to data will be critical to codifying approaches, quality assurance, and the dissemination of learnings—thus supporting more effective approaches to measuring outcomes, promoting equity, and informing resource allocation and policy.

REFERENCES

AAFP (American Academy of Family Physicians). 2019a. *The EveryONE Project tool kit.* https://www.aafp.org/patient-care/social-determinants-of-health/everyone-project/eop-tools.html (accessed May 22, 2019).

AAFP. 2019b. *Turning statistics into information: HealthLandsdcape.* https://www.healthlandscape.org (accessed April 15, 2019).

Abu-Saad, K., S. Avni, and O. Kalter-Leibovici. 2018. Health disparities monitoring in the U.S.: Lessons for monitoring efforts in Israel and other countries. *Israel Journal of Health Policy Research* 7(1):14.

AHA (American Hospital Association). 2019. *Sharing data, saving lives: The hospital agenda for interoperability.* https://www.aha.org/system/files/2019-01/Report01_18_19-Sharing-Data-Saving-Lives_FINAL.pdf (accessed May 22, 2019).

Alley, D. E., C. N. Asomugha, P. H. Conway, and D. M. Sanghavi. 2016. Accountable health communities—Addressing social needs through Medicare and Medicaid. *New England Journal of Medicine* 374(1):8–11.

Amarasingham, R., B. Kapoor, A. Karam, N. Nguyen, and B. Xie. 2018. *Using community partnerships to integrate health and social services for high-need, high-cost patients.* The Commonwealth Fund issue brief, January. https://www.commonwealthfund.org/sites/default/files/documents/___media_files_publications_issue_brief_2018_jan_amarasingham_integrating_health_social_services_high_need_high_cost_ib.pdf (accessed May 22, 2019).

Arons, A., S. DeSilvey, C. Fichtenberg, and L. Gottlieb. 2018. Documenting social determinants of health-related clinical activities using standardized medical vocabularies. *Journal of the American Medical Informatics Association Open* 2(1):81–88.

Auger, K. A., R. S. Kahn, J. M. Simmons, B. Huang, A. N. Shah, K. Timmons, and A. F. Beck. 2017. Using address information to identify hardships reported by families of children hospitalized with asthma. *Academic Pediatrics* 17(1):79–87.

Barrett, M., V. Combs, J. G. Su, K. Henderson, M. Tuffli, and AIR Louisville Collaborative. 2018. AIR Louisville: Addressing asthma with technology, crowdsourcing, cross-sector collaboration, and policy. *Health Affairs (Millwood)* 37(4):525–534.

Beam, A. L., and I. S. Kohane. 2018. Big data and machine learning in health care. *JAMA* 319(13):1317–1318.

Billioux, A., K. Verlander, S. Anthony, and D. Alley. 2017. *Standardized screening for health-related social needs in clinical settings: The accountable health communities screening tool.* Discussion Paper, National Academy of Medicine, Washington, DC. https://nam.edu/wp-content/uploads/2017/05/Standardized-Screening-for-Health-Related-Social-Needs-in-Clinical-Settings.pdf (accessed May 22, 2019).

Byhoff, E., A. J. Cohen, M. C. Hamati, J. Tatko, M. M. Davis, and R. Tipirneni. 2018. Screening for social determinants of health in Michigan health centers. *Journal of the American Board of Family Medicine* 30:418–427.

California Governor's Office of Planning and Research. 2018. *Precision medicine: An action plan for California.* http://opr.ca.gov/docs/20190107-Precision_Medicine_An_Action_Plan_for_California.pdf (accessed May 22, 2019).

Cantor, M. N., and L. Thorpe. 2018. Integrating data on social determinants of health into electronic health records. *Health Affairs (Millwood)* 37(4):585–590.

CARIN Alliance. 2019. *CARIN alliance.* https://www.carinalliance.com (accessed March 18, 2019).

CDC (Centers for Disease Control and Prevention). 2019. *Public health law.* https://www.cdc.gov/phlp/publications/topic/index.html (accessed April 15, 2019).

Char, D. S., N. H. Shah, and D. Magnus. 2018. Implementing machine learning in health care—Addressing ethical challenges. *New England Journal of Medicine* 378(11):979–981.

CMS (Centers for Medicare & Medicaid Services). 2019a. *Blue Button 2.0.* https://bluebutton.cms.gov/#overview (accessed February 21, 2019).

CMS. 2019b. *Medicare and Medicaid programs; Patient Protection and Affordable Care Act; interoperability and patient access for Medicare Advantage Organization and Medicaid managed care plans, state Medicaid agencies, CHIP agencies and CHIP managed care entities, issuers of qualified health plans in the federally-facilitated exchanges and health care providers.* Federal Register. https://www.federalregister.gov/documents/2019/03/04/2019-02200/medicare-and-medicaid-programs-patient-protection-and-affordable-care-act-interoperability-and (accessed May 22, 2019).

CMS. 2019c. *Promoting interoperability.* https://www.cms.gov/Regulations-and-Guidance/Legislation/EHRIncentivePrograms/index.html (accessed April 12, 2019).

Cookson, R., M. Asaria, S. Ali, R. Shaw, T. Doran, and P. Goldblatt. 2018. Health equity monitoring for healthcare quality assurance. *Social Science & Medicine* 198:148–156.

Dameff, C., B. Clay, and C. A. Longhurst. 2019. Personal health records: More promising in the smartphone era? *JAMA* 321(4):339–340.

Daniel, H., S. S. Bornstein, G. C. Kane, Health and Public Policy Committee of the American College of Physicians. 2018. Addressing social determinants to improve patient care and promote health equity: An American College of Physicians position paper. *Annals of Internal Medicine* 168(8):577–578.

Day, S., and M. Zweig. 2018. *2018 Year End Funding Report: Is digital health in a bubble?* In Rock Health: Reports. https://rockhealth.com/reports/2018-year-end-funding-report-is-digital-health-in-a-bubble (accessed April 15, 2019).

Freij, M., P. Dullabh, L. Hovey, J. Leonard, A. Card, and R. Dhopeshwarkar. 2018. *Incorporating social determinants of health in electronic health records: A qualitative study of perspectives on current practices among top vendors.* Report prepared for Assistant Secretary for Planning and Evaluation, U.S. Department of Health and Human Services. https://aspe.hhs.gov/system/files/pdf/259901/NORCSDH.pdf (accessed May 22, 2019).

Gangopadhyaya, A., G. M. Kenney, R. A. Burton, and J. Marks. 2018. *Medicaid work requirements in Arkansas.* The Urban Institute. https://www.urban.org/research/publication/medicaid-work-requirements-arkansas (accessed May 22, 2019).

Gold, R., A. Bruce, S. Cowburn, K. Dambrun, M. Dearing, M. Middendorf, N. Mossman, C. Hollombe, P. Mahr, G. Melgar, J. Davis, L. Gottlieb, and E. Cotrell. 2018. Adoption of social determinants of health EHR tools by community health centers. *Annals of Family Medicine* 16(5):399–407.

Gottlieb, L. M., and H. Alderwick. 2019. Integrating social and medical care: Could it worsen health and increase inequity. *Annals of Family Medicine* 17(1):77–81.

Gottlieb, L. M., D. E. Francis, and A. F. Beck. 2018. Uses and misuses of patient- and neighborhood-level social determinants of health data. *The Permanente Journal* 22:18-078.

Hanak, M. 2018. *The numbers tell a story: How to use data to achieve health equity.* Improvement Blog: Institute for Healthcare Improvement. March 27. http://www.ihi.org/communities/blogs/the-numbers-tell-a-story-how-to-use-data-to-achieve-health-equity (accessed May 22, 2019).

Hanna-Attisha, M., J. LaChance, R. C. Sadler, and A. Champney Schnepp. 2016. Elevated blood lead levels in children associated with the Flint drinking water crisis: A spatial analysis of risk and public health response. *American Journal of Public Health* 106(2):283–290.

HHS (U.S. Department of Health and Human Services). 2018. *Request for information on modifying HIPAA rules to improve coordinated care.* https://www.federalregister.gov/documents/2018/12/14/2018-27162/request-for-information-on-modifying-hipaa-rules-to-improve-coordinated-care (accessed April 15, 2019).

HL7 International. 2019. *Argo-2018-projects.* http://argonautwiki.hl7.org/index.php?title=Argo-2018-Projects (accessed March 18, 2019).

Illinois Department of Human Services. 2013. *Establishing governance for health and human services interoperability initiatives: A handbook for states.* https://www.acf.hhs.gov/sites/default/files/assets/establishing_governance_for_hhs_handbook_508compliant_final.pdf (accessed May 22, 2019).

IOM (Institute of Medicine). 2009. *Beyond the HIPAA privacy rule: Enhancing privacy, improving health through research.* Washington, DC: The National Academies Press.

IOM. 2013. *Digital data improvement priorities for continuous learning in health and health care: Workshop summary.* Washington, DC: The National Academies Press.

IOM. 2014. *Capturing social and behavioral domains and measures in electronic health records: Phase 2.* Washington, DC: The National Academies Press.

Kasthurirathne, S. N., J. R. Vest, N. Menachemi, P. K. Halverson, and S. J. Grannis. 2018. Assessing the capacity of social determinants of health data to augment predictive models identifying patients in need of wraparound social services. *Journal of the American Medical Informatics Association* 25(1):47–53.

Messer, L. C., B. A. Laraia, J. S. Kaufman, J. Eyster, C. Holzman, J. Culhane, I. Elo, J. G. Burke, and P. O'Campo. 2006. The development of a standardized neighborhood deprivation index. *Journal of Urban Health* 83(6):1041–1062.

MyHealth Access Network. 2019. *Accountable health communities—Route 66 Consortium.* https://myhealthaccess.net/ahc (accessed April 15, 2019).

NAAAA (National Association of Area Agencies on Aging). 2015. *Information technology in area agencies on aging—Report from the 2015 National AAA Survey.* https://www.n4a.org/Files/UPDATE%20Information%20Technology%20in%20AAAs%20-%20Report%20from%202015%20National%20Survey.pdf (accessed May 22, 2019).

NACHC (National Association of Community Health Centers). 2019. *PRAPARE implementation and action toolkit.* http://www.nachc.org/research-and-data/prapare/toolkit (accessed May 22, 2019).

NACHC, Association of Asian Pacific Community Health Organizations, Oregon Primary Care Assocation, and Institute for Alternative Futures. 2016. *Accelerating strategies to address the social determinants of health—Protocol for responding to and addessing patients' assets, risks, and experiences.* http://www.nachc.org/wp-content/uploads/2016/07/PRAPARE-Abstract-4-20-16.pdf (accessed May 22, 2019).

NASDOH (National Alliance to Impact the Social Determinants of Health). 2019. *Identifying social risk and needs in health care.* http://www.nasdoh.org/wp-content/uploads/2019/01/NASDOH-Social-Risks-Issue-Brief.pdf (access May 22, 2019).

National Interoperability Collaborative. 2019. *Partnerships, programs, and platforms.* https://www.academyhealth.org/sites/default/files/partnerships_programs_platforms_april2019.pdf (acessed May 22, 2019).

Navathe, A. S., F. Zhong, V. J. Lei, F. Y. Chang, M. Sordo, M. Topaz, S. B. Navathe, R. A. Rocha, and L. Zhou. 2018. Hospital readmission and social risk factors identified from physician notes. *Health Services Research* 53(2):1110–1136.

NC DHHS (North Carolina Department of Health and Human Services). 2019. NCCARE 360. https://www.ncdhhs.gov/about/department-initiatives/healthy-opportunities/nccare360 (accessed June 6, 2019).

NCCBH (National Council for Community Behavioral Healthcare). 2012. *HIT adoption and readiness for meaningful use in community behavioral health—report on the 2012 National Council Survey.* https://www.thenationalcouncil.org/wp-content/uploads/2012/10/HIT-Survey-Full-Report.pdf (accessed May 22, 2019).

ONC (The Office of the National Coordinator for Health Information Technology). 2014. *Blue Button fact sheet.* https://www.healthit.gov/sites/default/files/blue-button-fact-sheet-2014-feb_0.pdf (accessed May 22, 2019).

ONC. 2016. *Update on the adoption of the health information technology and related efforts to facilitate the electronic use and exchange of health information.* Report to Congress, February. https://www.healthit.gov/sites/default/files/Attachment_1_-_2-26-16_RTC_Health_IT_Progress.pdf (accessed May 22, 2019).

ONC. 2018. *Federal health architecture (FHS).* https://www.healthit.gov/topic/onc-hitech-programs/federal-health-architecture-fha (accessed April 15, 2019).

ONC. 2019. *Office-based physician electronic health record adoption.* http:///quickstats/pages/physician-ehr-adoption-trends.php (accessed June 6. 2019).

Onie, R. D., R. Lavizzo-Mourey, T. H. Lee, J. S. Marks, and R. J. Perla. 2018. Integrating social needs into health care: A twenty-year case study of adaptation and diffusion. *Health Affairs* 37(2):240–247.

Pew Research Center. 2019. *Demographics of mobile device ownership and adoption in the United States*. https://www.pewinternet.org/fact-sheet/mobile (accessed April 15, 2019).

Price, W. N., 2nd, and I. G. Cohen. 2019. Privacy in the age of medical big data. *Nature Medicine* 25(1):37–43.

Raghupathi, W., and V. Raghupathi. 2014. Big data analytics in healthcare: Promise and potential. *Health Information Science and Systems* 2(3):PMC4341817.

Reisman, M. 2017. EHRs: The challenge of making electronic data usable and interoperable. *Pharmacy and Therapeutics* 42(9):572–575.

Richards, C. L., M. F. Iademarco, D. Atkinson, R. W. Pinner, P. Yoon, W. R. Mac Kenzie, B. Lee, J. R. Qualters, and T. R. Frieden. 2017. Advances in public health surveillance and information dissemination at the Centers for Disease Control and Prevention. *Public Health Reports* 132(4):403–410.

Robert Grahm Center. 2019. *Community oriented primary care (COPC) curriculum*. https://www.graham-center.org/rgc/maps-data-tools/tools/copc.html (accessed March 20, 2019).

Rucker, D. 2018. *Achieving the interoperability promise of 21st Century Cures*. Health Affairs blog. https://www.healthaffairs.org/do/10.1377/hblog20180618.138568/full (accessed May 22, 2019).

Rudowitz, R., M. Musumeci, and C. Hall. 2019. *February state data for Medicaid work requirements in Arkansas*. Kaiser Family Foundation. https://www.kff.org/medicaid/issue-brief/state-data-for-medicaid-work-requirements-in-arkansas (accessed May 22, 2019).

Shah, A. K., J. Zhao, S. Mullainathan, and E. Shafir. 2018. Money in the mental lives of the poor. *Social Cognition* 36(1):4–19.

SIREN (Social Interventions Research and Evaluation Network). 2019. *The Gravity Project*. https://sirenetwork.ucsf.edu/TheGravityProject (accessed April 15, 2019).

TAMU (Texas A&M University). 2019. *TAMU geoservices*. http://geoservices.tamu.edu (accessed April 15, 2019).

Town Hall Ventures. 2019. *What we do—Town Hall Ventures*. https://www.townhallventures.com/what-we-do (accessed April 15, 2019).

Washington, V., K. DeSalvo, F. Mostashari, and D. Blumenthal. 2017. The HITECH era and the path forward. *New England Journal of Medicine* 377(10):901–904.

Wyman, O., and SeaChange Capital Partners. 2017. *A national imperative: Joining forces to strengthen human services in America in 2018*. Alliance for Strong Families and Communities and American Public Human Services Association. https://www.alliance1.org/web/resources/pubs/national-imperative-joining-forces-strengthen-human-services-america.aspx (accessed April 15, 2019).

5

Financing Social Care

This chapter begins with a general overview of current health care and social care financing in the United States. Next, five financial barriers are discussed along with promising approaches to dealing with those barriers and financing the integration of health care and social care. The chapter concludes with the committee's findings.

CURRENT HEALTH AND SOCIAL CARE FINANCING

Health Care Spending

In 2017, an estimated $3.5 trillion was spent in the United States for health care services, or 18 percent of the U.S. gross domestic product (GDP) (CMS, 2017b), a higher percentage of GDP spent on health care than any of the other 34 Organisation for Economic Co-operation and Development (OECD) member countries (Squires and Anderson, 2015). Sources for this spending include publicly and privately funded health insurance ($2.6 trillion, 74.7 percent of national health expenditure [NHE]), out-of-pocket expenses for individuals ($365.3 billion, 10.5 percent of NHE), other third-party payers ($352.8 billion, 10.1 percent of NHE), and investments such as noncommercial research and structures and equipment ($163.9 billion, 4.7 percent of NHE) (see Table 5-1).

Historically, U.S. health care spending has increased faster than the general U.S. economy, and it is projected to continue to do so for the foreseeable future, driven in part by increases in the price of health care services, worsening health status, and an aging population that is expected

TABLE 5-1
National Health Expenditures (NHEs) in Billions $USD, Aggregate and per Capita Amounts, Share of Gross Domestic Product (GDP), and Average Annual Growth from Previous Year Shown, by Source of Funds, Selected Calendar Years 2013–2026

Source of Funds	2013	2015	2016	2017	2018	2020	2026
NHE	$2,879.0	$3,200.8	$3,337.2	$3,489.2	$3,675.3	$4,090.9	$5,696.2
Health consumption expenditures	2,725.9	3,047.1	3,179.8	3,325.4	3,504.3	3,901.7	5,437.1
Out of pocket	325.2	339.3	352.5	365.3	379.8	417.3	555.3
Health insurance	2,087.8	2,382.8	2,486.8	2,607.3	2,755.2	3,075.6	4,351.9
Private	946.4	1,068.8	1,123.4	1,186.6	1,244.1	1,348.8	1,776.0
Medicare	590.2	648.8	672.1	705.8	748.1	873.1	1,366.0
Medicaid	445.4	544.1	565.5	582.0	622.0	696.4	996.2
Federal	256.9	343.1	358.1	360.4	385.8	429.4	613.0
State and local	188.5	201.0	207.5	221.7	236.2	267.0	383.2
Other health insurance and public health	105.9	121.1	125.8	132.8	141.1	157.3	213.8
Other third-party payers	312.9	325.0	340.5	352.8	369.2	408.8	529.8
Investment	153.1	153.7	157.4	163.9	171.1	189.2	259.2
NHE as percent of GDP	17.2%	17.7%	17.9%	18.0%	18.2%	18.4%	19.7%

SOURCE: Copyrighted and published by Project HOPE/Health Affairs as Gigi A. Cuckler, Andrea M. Sisko, John A. Poisal, et al. "National Health Expenditure Projections, 2017–26: Despite Uncertainty, Fundamentals Primarily Drive Spending Growth." *Health Affairs (Millwood)*. 2018, Vol. 37, No. 3, pp. 482–492, exhibit 1. The published article is archived and available online at www.healthaffairs.org. Adapted with permission from Project HOPE/Health Affairs.

to consume more services (Cuckler et al., 2018). By 2026, health spending is projected to amount to $5.7 trillion, or nearly 20 percent of GDP (Cuckler et al., 2018). Per capita health care expenses are also projected to rise from $10,723.50 in 2017 to $16,167.60 in 2026 (Cuckler et al., 2018).

The high rate of growth of U.S. health care costs creates budget pressures for employers, public officials, and competing public services. Consumers also face "underinsurance," which may negatively affect health outcomes. Underinsurance includes increased cost sharing and limited coverage benefits that occur as employers respond to these price increases (Schoen et al., 2005). Health care spending growth in excess of the general economy also may harm the international competitiveness of the U.S. private sector (Gara, 2018).

Social Care Spending

Spending estimates within the U.S. social services sector are less well defined than those for health care. International economic analyses (e.g., among OECD countries) define social services as public and private spending, including spending for cash transfers and tax treatments for programs in old age, incapacity-related (disability) payments, active labor market policies, unemployment, and housing, among other categories. By this definition, social spending in the United States approaches that of health care spending but accounts for a considerably lower percentage of GDP than social spending in other countries (see Figure 1-1).

Health care and social care spending are both related to health outcomes. OECD countries that spend a higher proportion of their GDP on social services than on health care have better health outcomes than those that do not (see Chapter 1 and also Bradley and Taylor, 2013; Rubin et al., 2016). This also holds true within the United States, as states with higher ratios of social-to-health spending appear to have better health outcomes than those with lower ratios (Bradley et al., 2016). Among the OECD industrialized countries, the United States has the lowest ratio of social-to-health spending: for every $1 spent on health care in the United States, about $0.90 is spent on social services, while in OECD countries, for every $1 spent on health care, an average of $2 is spent on social services (see Figure 1-1).

According to a 2016 RAND Europe report, U.S. social care spending (e.g., on unemployment and housing) is lower than it is in other member countries in the OECD, and spending on old age (e.g., pensions and home-help and residential services) is higher than comparative OECD countries (see Table 5-2). It appears that as the health care sector responds to growing evidence of the importance of the social determinants of health (SDOH) with increasing integration of social care, the challenges of financing the

TABLE 5-2
Size of Individual Social Spending Categories, with Examples, as a Share of Overall Social Expenditure (2011 Values)

Category	Example	United States	OECD Average	EU15 Average
Old age	Pensions, home-help and residential services for the elderly	66.1%	50.4%	48.9%
Survivors	Pensions and funeral payments	4.4%	6.2%	6.7%
Incapacity-related	Care services, disability benefits, workers' injury compensation, employee sickness payments	11.7%	14.6%	14.8%
Family	Child allowances and credits, child care support, income support during leave, sole parent payments	4.5%	13.3%	12.4%
Active labor market policies	Employment services and incentives, training, direct job creation, start-up incentives	0.8%	2.8%	3.9%
Unemployment	Unemployment compensation, early retirement for labor market reasons	5.0%	5.2%	7.4%
Housing	Housing allowances, rent subsidies	1.9%	2.7%	2.0%
Other	Cash benefits to low-income households, food subsidies, other social services	5.6%	4.9%	3.8%

SOURCE: Adapted from Rubin et al., 2016. Reprinted with permission from the RAND Corporation.

integration of social care with health care are not a matter of how social care spending is divided among different categories, but of definition and rebalancing. These challenges are discussed in the next section.

BARRIERS TO FINANCING THE INTEGRATION OF SOCIAL CARE AND PROMISING SOLUTIONS

Substantial barriers to the financing of social and health care integration remain. Five primary challenges, with promising solutions, are discussed below: (1) definitions of health care, (2) payment reforms, (3) accountability, (4) fragmented financing for dually eligible beneficiaries, and (5) a lack of administrative capacity for social care providers.

Legal Definitions of Health Care

The first challenge to financing the integration of social care and health care has to do with the origins of insurance and medical care. Due to the size and expense of treating medical events, most health care financing is by a third party—either using an insurance model or public financing (Cuckler et al., 2018). Third-party financing, in turn, requires a definition, either via contract or statute, of what services are covered and which are excluded. Furthermore, both public and private coverage standards are based on an exclusively medical model of care; this drives the definition of what constitutes medical care and is to be paid for by third parties (Flexner, 1910).

Commercial insurance contracts set standards on covered health care services. These standards typically refer to covered services as being those deemed "medically necessary" by an ordering physician (provider), based on the standards of accepted medical practice. Public financing sources—Medicaid and Medicare—also require services to be medically necessary and use evolving definitions of what can be covered if medically necessary. Within this statutory framework, Medicare policies are set by federal payment rules and to some extent by "local coverage determinations" made by a Medicare fiscal intermediary or carrier. Medicaid coverage policy parameters are also set by federal regulations, but states have flexibility to adopt optional benefits and to define, particularly with respect to adults, the "amount, scope, and duration" (42 CFR 438.3) of a covered benefit. In addition, Medicaid rules offer health plans additional authority to voluntarily cover additional services (including non-medical services) for Medicaid beneficiaries whenever a health plan determines those services to be of value to the individual, although the cost of the services cannot be factored into the payment rates (42 CFR 438.3).

Financing the integration of social care into the medical model of care requires defining activities of social care (defined by the committee as awareness, adjustment, assistance, and alignment; see Chapter 2 for a description of the committee's five activities involved in integrating social care into health care) within the constructs of current definitions of medical care (Miller et al., 2010). Federal and state governments are exploring creating the flexibility to broaden the definition of what constitutes medical care in order to make it possible to finance the integration and provision of some types of social care into health care. Most of these increased flexibility efforts are occurring in Medicaid, which pays for the care of people with greater needs. The extent of this increased flexibility is evolving through both state plan definitions (the state plan is the "agreement" between the states and the Centers for Medicare & Medicaid Services [CMS] on what populations and services will be covered in that state) and managed care authorities. The federal government has the authority to allow states to pay for some care and services that otherwise would not be permissible to cover with federal Medicaid funds through both home and community-based waivers and more comprehensive waiver authority. The key areas of current flexibility in Medicaid are identified below.

Medicaid State Plan Authority

Under Medicaid states have the discretion to define the scope of benefits they will offer, subject to federal guidelines. Some Medicaid benefits allow states to incorporate aspects of social care into the standard operation of their Medicaid program, broadly or for a targeted population. Notably, various activities, including assessing needs and providing linkages to services that address those needs, such as homelessness and food assistance, can be financed through Medicaid by incorporating these activities in the state's definition of case management and health home services.[1] In addition, state plan services relating to home- and community-based long-term services also can incorporate a broad range of non-medical services, such as supportive housing services, employment services, and home modifications.

Medicaid Managed Care

As of September 2018, 39 states and the District of Columbia, which together cover about two-thirds of all Medicaid beneficiaries, had contracted with managed care organizations (MCOs) to deliver some or all of their Medicaid-funded services (Kaiser Family Foundation, 2018, 2019). States have made different decisions about which Medicaid benefits are administered by MCOs ("carved in") and which are administered through Medicaid fee-for-service ("carved out"). The potential for innovation by Medicaid health plans in this area is substantial—with funding from the state, accountabilities, and guidance on their limitations, plan administrators can make decisions about what the best use of their premium dollars is.

MCOs are obligated to provide care management, which includes the authority for MCOs to use their Medicaid funding to identify social care needs and to link people to available services. In addition, MCOs can use their Medicaid funds to pay for social care as "in lieu of" services or as "value added" services (e.g., to provide medically tailored meals for a homebound individual or an air conditioner for a severely asthmatic child) (Bachrach et al., 2018). State Medicaid agency contracts can encourage (through procurement processes or payment incentives) or require MCOs to undertake these activities, and some states require MCOs to contract with existing community-based organizations to provide services such as ombudsman (advocacy) services, nursing home eligibility assessments, and care management (CHCS/ACAP, 2018; Super et al., 2018).

[1] Case management is described in Section 1915(g)(2) in the Social Security Act and home health services in Section 1946 of the Act.

Furthermore, state Medicaid agencies have flexibility in allowing some social care to qualify as quality improvement activities in the calculation of the numerator of the medical loss ratio of MCOs.

To the extent that MCOs are at risk for health care costs, they have a financial incentive to make investments in social care to lower the rates of use of high-cost medical services. However, modifications in rate-setting methodologies, risk adjustments, and incentives often are needed to address the so-called premium slide, which can serve as a disincentive for plans to make social care investments. This term refers to the phenomenon whereby plans that invest in effective interventions that result in lower rates of use of high-cost care may be faced with a rate reduction the next time that rates are reset (California Health Care Foundation, 2018). Premium slide is not exclusive to activities addressing social needs; it can occur when plans are successful in being cost effective and efficient with health care dollars and is a risk with new payment models outside of fee-for-service.

Four practices can be employed by state Medicaid agencies with their contracted plans to accelerate the integration of social care into the health care setting: (1) using value-based payments to support provider investment in social interventions; (2) using incentives and withholds to encourage plan investment in social interventions; (3) integrating efforts to address social issues into quality improvement activities; and (4) rewarding plans through higher rates for effective investments in social interventions (Bachrach et al., 2018). McGinnis and colleagues, however, reviewed Medicaid agency contracts with their managed care plans and concluded that although there is a growing focus on the SDOH in state-managed care contracts, most states do not provide details on how MCOs can use flexibilities under federal law to provide services that address the SDOH and, furthermore, that payment incentives linked to these determinants are not yet commonplace (CHCS/ACAP, 2018).

Medicaid Waivers

States have the opportunity to innovate in Medicaid under specific agreements with CMS called waivers (Shrank et al., 2018). Two types of waivers—1915(c) and 1115—can offer state Medicaid programs additional, substantial flexibility and, potentially, funding for social care. The more targeted authority is available under section 1915(c) waivers, which authorize Medicaid spending on home and community-based services for people who need long-term care (CMS, 2015). More comprehensive section 1115 demonstration waiver authority—that can extend beyond people who need long-term care—has also been used to help finance social care interventions for Medicaid beneficiaries. Under various state waiver programs, some states and their contracted Medicaid plans are experimenting aggressively with paying for specific social services, such as employment supports and housing tenancy (Shrank et al., 2018). Additionally, social services provided in the context of delivering health care are also funded through other mechanisms federally and at state levels and are discussed further below in the section on accountability (the concepts of "braiding and blending").

Some states are making financing the integration of social care a priority (Bachrach et al., 2016). For example, North Carolina's 1115 demonstration waiver authorizes the state to use Medicaid payment for a defined set of services relating to priority areas—food insecurity, housing instability, transportation barriers, interpersonal violence, and toxic stress as part of regional pilots. Working closely with MCOs, the effectiveness of these services to improve health outcomes and decrease cost will be tested (NC DHHS, 2018). The North Carolina waiver requires a summative independent evaluation—as required for all 1115 waivers—and a rapid-cycle assessment process for efficacy testing. This second feature is notable because the utility of formal evaluations varies substantially.

The Oregon Health Authority uses coordinated care organizations (CCOs) through its 1115 Medicaid demonstration waiver authority. CCOs are expected to pay for what the states refer to as "flexible services" that can provide housing supports and assistance with food and other social resources (Alderwick et al., 2019; CMS, 2017b). In these arrangements, the state plays a critical role in providing guidance, direction, flexibility, and accountability for plans and providers.

A review of evaluations of Medicaid demonstrations from eight states with high-demonstration expenditures that varied in the number of years the demonstrations had been in effect and by geography found that the evaluations had substantial limitations that "affected their usefulness in informing policy decisions" (GAO, 2018). Efforts to improve the usefulness of state- and federal-led evaluations are under way.

CMS Guidance to States

CMS guidance to states on state plan and managed care options and its willingness to approve waiver authority to support social care are also critical. Although such guidance has historically been limited, the 2016 CMS managed care regulations provide some clarity. Still, however, questions remain as to what social care activities can be financed with Medicaid dollars. Machledt states that the regulation encourages Medicaid agencies to financially incentivize health plans to address social risks by allowing certain non-clinical services to be included as covered services when calculating the capitated rate and medical loss ratios (Machledt, 2017). The issue of how to account for the additional costs of these additional social needs integration benefits remains to be worked out in practice, and the extent to which the benefits are self-financing depends on how returns are calculated (see below).

Medicare Innovations

Medicare has begun to follow Medicaid's lead in this work and has recently given guidance to the health plans it contracts with in the Medicare Advantage Program regarding particular non-medical services that can be considered supplemental benefits available to all or a subset of the plan's enrollees. These non-medical benefits, made permissible under the CHRONIC portion of the Bipartisan Budget Act of 2018,[2] are to be coupled with changes in rate-setting methodology for the plans that provide them (Wynne and Horowitz, 2018). The goal of the expanded supplemental benefits is to meet the needs of chronically ill Medicare Advantage enrollees. Early indications are that Medicare Advantage plan organizations are generally interested in the increased flexibility (Long-Term Quality Alliance, 2018). As is the case with Medicaid, it remains to be seen whether Medicare Advantage plans need more specific government direction. While the legislation enables Medicare Advantage Plans to cover some social care for beneficiaries, traditional Medicare plans still largely do not support social care provision.

There is a call for reforming the Medicare Advantage competitive bidding process. The original goal of the process was for private health plans to demonstrate care coordination and high-quality care while providing enhanced benefits for beneficiaries and saving money for taxpayers, as compared with traditional Medicare, which is fee-for-service. Research indicates that the current Medicare Advantage bidding structure does not promote competition allowing plans to overbid, retain the dollars, and not pass the savings to their enrollees (Lieberman et al., 2018).

Health Care Payment Reform

A second challenge to financing social care integration is the method of provider payment, which can have a substantial dampening or accelerating effect on the integration of social care into the health care setting.

Health care providers have generally been paid for their services on a fee-for-service basis, where Medicare rates are a point of reference for both Medicaid and commercial insurers. The shortcomings of fee-for-service

[2] Public Law 123, 115th Cong. (February 9, 2018). https://www.congress.gov/115/plaws/publ123/PLAW-115publ123.pdf (accessed May 23, 2019).

and Medicare rate setting compensation have been well documented (Laugesen, 2017), and they include incentivizing providers to produce volume over value and to value technical excellence over services of cognition and coordination (Bodenheimer et al., 2007). Services of cognition and coordination include various activities of social care integration, such as screening for social needs (awareness) or connecting patients to social care providers (assistance); these activities have not been reimbursable, and thus they are not incentivized under traditional fee-for-service compensation methods. While the overall movement in provider payment reform has been away from fee-for-service toward value-based payment, it is important to explicitly define and acknowledge social care activities as well as expand on which individuals can bill for such services. Doing so provides resources for social care integration in the near term and may inform and foster more advanced payment models. Within the fee-for-service compensation methods, adding billing codes or modifying existing codes in the fee schedule to allow providers to bill for care coordination activities may be one opportunity to finance social care (Improving Care for Medicare Beneficiaries with Chronic Conditions, Committee on Finance, U.S. Senate, 2015). For example, Medicare Chronic Care Management Services codes that physicians and other qualified health care providers are eligible to bill also allow for other members of the care team to provide services under the billing providers' general supervision (CMS, 2016). This expansion of billing codes and explicit inclusion of other qualified health care providers (such as licensed social workers) in being able to contribute to billable services is a key step to enabling health care systems to invest in social care providers.

With the passage of the Patient Protection and Affordable Care Act of 2010[3] (ACA) and the establishment of the Center for Medicare & Medicaid Innovation (CMMI; a center within CMS), efforts by Medicare to reform provider payments accelerated. While work on population health financing was pursued at CMMI, particularly in state innovation models (Kissam et al., 2019) and the seminal work of the Accountable Communities for Health project (Alley et al., 2016), that work is best considered capacity planning and payment model development. CMMI provider payment models, once they have been developed, are to be tested and, if successful, implemented. They can be categorized in the areas of accountable care, service bundles, and comprehensive primary care. The committee found descriptions in the literature of the work of accountable care organizations for commercially insured and Medicare populations to integrate social care into health care settings, but the number and comprehensiveness of those descriptions

[3] Public Law 148, 111th Cong. (March 23, 2010). https://www.congress.gov/111/plaws/publ148/PLAW-111publ148.pdf (accessed May 23, 2019).

were substantially smaller than in the literature for Medicaid, presumably reflecting the lower incidence of needs in those populations. Value-based payment models appear to serve a necessary, but not sufficient, mechanism for integrating social care into health care by creating stronger financial incentives for providers to focus on care coordination, prevention, and outcomes (McWilliams et al., 2016). However, there is little evidence to indicate that actual integration or savings from these models are being redirected to financing social care (Chaiyachati et al., 2016; KPMG, 2018).

Medicare efforts have led to similar movements by Medicaid and commercial payers. This section will not address the relative efficacy of the payment reform models in general but will focus instead on efforts in Medicaid—where the care of the population with the highest social needs is financed—to use provider payment reform to facilitate integration and payment of social care.

State Medicaid payment reform efforts do not generally require special waivers or authority from CMMI, although some states have benefited by additional waiver funding (e.g., from the Delivery System Reform Incentive Payment Program) or CMMI support. States have established payment reforms in all three CMMI categories—comprehensive primary care, service bundles, and accountable care—particularly through existing Medicaid managed care contracts where MCOs are directed to implement the payment reforms.

There is some evidence from the ACA-initiated health homes that Medicaid provider payment reform efforts in the areas of comprehensive primary care have facilitated enhanced integration of social care into the health care setting (ASPE, 2018). Evaluations of the effects of other large state-led Medicaid comprehensive primary care payment reform efforts on the integration of social care could not be located.

The most comprehensive Medicaid provider payment reform efforts have been in the area of accountable care, often implemented in tandem with delivery reform waivers. In theory, a group of providers of care to Medicaid beneficiaries, held accountable for population health outcomes, financially incentivized through a reconciliation to a total budget for costs and given the flexibility of new covered services, will spend more time assessing the social needs of their patients and arranging for those needs to be met. Perhaps the most mature programmatic example of this is Oregon's CCO model (MN DHS, 2018; Stock and Goldberg, 2017), but other examples include efforts in Minnesota, Colorado, and Vermont, among other states (CHCS, 2018). More recently, Massachusetts has adopted a variation of this approach (MassHealth, 2018).

The models differ considerably in their design details—including the role of existing managed care organizations, methods of payment to provider groups related to quality and other accountability measures, guidance on covered benefits, and partnerships with community-based organizations. There is no research available that indicates which, if any, of these accountable care models are, in fact, achieving more social care integration, let alone whether that integration is improving health. Instead, practitioners—states and providers—are engaged in rapid cycles of experimentation, often facilitated by for-profit and nonprofit technical assistance providers (Crumley and Marlise, 2018). How to discern, disseminate, and deploy these lessons from payment reform remains a substantial policy challenge, not only in the realm of social care integration, but also for provider payment reform efforts in general.

A final provider payment model involves salaried providers of health care—whether in fully integrated systems of care such as the Veterans Health Administration and Kaiser Permanente or in Medicare and Medicaid capitated programs such as the Programs of All-Inclusive Care for the Elderly (PACE)—that may be less susceptible to the incentives of fee-for-service medicine that make the work of integrating social care more challenging.

For all three of these models there are examples of attempts to attend to the social care needs of patients (Meyer, 2012). However, in addition to the capital costs required to build a fully integrated salaried model of care, the constraints on patient choice called for in these models have long been thought to limit their broader attractiveness and applicability (Meyer, 2012).

Accountability

A third challenge to financing the integration of social care and health care is at once fundamental and complex: For what services and outcomes are plans, health care providers, and social service providers accountable, and how will that accountability be defined and measured?

Traditional inputs for accountability in health care are the activities of providers, and these activities are generally measured through the use of disease classification (e.g., with the *International Statistical Classification of Diseases and Related Health Problems, 10th Revision* [ICD-10]) and procedure codes (e.g., Current Procedures Terminology [CPT]). These codes are specified in great detail, reflecting the need for providers to receive reimbursement for the care they deliver and the importance of using these codes as part of risk-adjusting in pay-for-value settings.

In keeping with the traditional medical model of health care, neither social care activities (awareness, adjustment, assistance, and alignment) nor social risks and social needs are well documented. However, systems such as ICD-10, LOINC, SNOMED, and CPT now include new disease classification codes (e.g., Z55–Z65 in the ICD-10 system) as a way to begin to measure activities associated with social care. The codes include social risk factors, such as problems related to education and literacy, employment, housing and economic circumstances, and social environment (Arons et al., 2018; Gottlieb et al., 2016). However, while these codes are available, some reports suggest that they are not yet frequently used (AHA, 2018; Torres et al., 2017). Furthermore, there is no similar coding system that providers can use to document and measure the delivery of social needs services. States, plans, and providers who may be at financial risk for the cost of care for populations will need improved ways to assess the accountability of social care delivery. As noted in Chapter 4, efforts are under way to develop documentation standards across coding vocabularies used in electronic health records to develop consensus on key concepts; these efforts should improve interoperability in this area.

Another accountability issue centers broadly on outputs and outcomes: For what measures—both general measures and those related to social care integration—are providers and plans to be held accountable? Accountability measures, even in the most mature Medicaid accountable care programs, have not been tightly focused; instead, they have included a broad array of measures across several domains with great variety among the states (CHCS, 2017). State Medicaid agencies are developing their own accountability measures dealing with social care. As with payment models, there is no evidence about which measures are more effective or about how they should be implemented and enforced. Specific to the topic of this report, the most important question may be: Is a particular measurement focused on the activities of social care necessary, or would the adoption of broader outcome measures encourage the development of effective integration practices in an attempt to succeed at those measures? Providers, states, plans, Medicaid agencies, and their advisers, in the absence of definitive research evidence, continue to try and improve in their measurement efforts.

To the extent that providers should be held accountable not only for relative improvement but also for performance compared to a standard, how should their performance be adjusted for characteristics and population risks that are beyond the providers' control? This question is not unique to the challenge of integrating social care and health care, but developing standard practices to answer it will facilitate integration efforts. Research has found that adjusting for additional patient characteristics—including socioeconomic position; race, ethnicity, and cultural context; gender; social relationships; and residential and community context—narrowed performance differences between those practices that cared for more socially and medical complex patients and those that cared for fewer complex patients (Joynt et al., 2017). The same researchers expressed concern that inadequate clinical and social risk adjustment may lead to payments being directed away from those practices serving poorer and sicker patients because of perceived poor performance, even though the "poor performance" may not reflect the true quality or efficiency of care. As such, practices that care for a large proportion of high-cost, sicker, poorer, or otherwise vulnerable patients may not have the resources to care for the population and may be forced to avoid caring for them, which may worsen disparities (Roberts et al., 2018).

Notably, the conclusion in a National Academies of Sciences, Engineering, and Medicine (the National Academies) report on the research evidence for adjustments to Medicare value-based payment programs for social risk factors is directly applicable to this issue:

> The committee supports four goals of accounting for social risk factors in Medicare payment programs: reducing disparities in access, quality, and outcomes; improving quality and efficient care delivery for all patients; fair and accurate reporting; and compensating health plans and providers fairly. These goals would best be achieved through payment based on performance measure scores adjusted for social risk factors (or adjusting payment directly for these risk factors) when combined with public reporting stratified by patient characteristics within reporting units. (NASEM, 2017, p. 16)

The committee that authored that report could find no evidence of the adoption of these types of risk adjustment practices within Medicaid outcome measurement efforts (NASEM, 2017).

Integrating social care into health care will further accelerate the evolution of the use of outcome-based contracting. In particular, while the complexities of developing comparable outcome measures for health care providers are noted above, the use of outcomes-based contracting for social care organizations is nascent.

Even if social services accountability measures can be established and appropriately adjusted for factors beyond the control of providers, the possibility remains that the benefits of a managed care organization or at-risk provider investing in efforts to integrate social care needs will accrue only at a later date or to another party, such as the educational or child welfare systems (Taylor and Nichols, 2018). This "wrong pockets problem" often is an issue for children's services, and it is exacerbated when individuals enter and exit the accountable entity's population, whether that entity is a provider, a health plan, or a geographic community (Urban Institute, 2017).

The immediate cause of entry and exit from a population often is program eligibility, or "churn," which can be caused by a failure to comply with administrative requirements or the nature of the requirements themselves. Although some consider churn to be in the financial interests of the funding agency (usually Medicaid) because it reduces, if temporarily, the number of covered lives and thus payments to plans and providers, the costs of administration and interrupted care have been estimated to outweigh any savings (Swartz et al., 2015), giving rise to federal and state policies promoting continuous eligibility for Medicaid enrollees.

Even with continuous eligibility, the returns for investing in the integration of social care can accrue to other parties. Moreover, Medicaid is statutorily forbidden from paying for social services such as housing or food. As a result, other sources of funding are needed. The "braiding and blending" of public sources of funding to pay for prioritized social services creates a local environment where "assistance" and "alignment" activities to social care integration are more likely to happen; for example, it makes sense to screen for housing needs in a health care setting if options for meeting the needs exist and can be accessed (Soper, 2017). The "braided" approach may have important consequences; for instance, the human capital required to support multiple sources can make social care programs more difficult to initiate and sustain (Gottlieb et al., 2019).

Even with more effective blending of funding sources, the horizon for returns on social investments often remains long and the wrong pockets problem persists. This is a structural challenge and has been historically a rationale for public-sector accountability and action. Geographically exclusive accountable care organizations, such as those in Oregon's program, have the advantage of a longer time horizon for expecting returns, because they will not be losing population to another provider, but their existence comes with the economic risk of monopoly provider status. Social impact bonds also have been proposed and implemented in certain circumstances to make accountability for performance more direct and clearer than is the case with public-sector taxation and budgeting. However, the use of these bonds in health care settings has been limited (Stoesz, 2014). Some researchers have suggested that social care financing should be considered a public good and have theorized about the use of structures of collective governance, investment, and accountability to address the problems of wrong pocket, free rider, and long-term returns for investments in social care integration and more upstream investment in pediatric populations, which are larger than a single provider but smaller than governmental organizations (Taylor and Nichols, 2018).

Others see the traditional hospital role of large civic institutions as the basis for such a collective structure. The ACA imposed clearer obligations on nonprofit hospitals to justify their tax status in annual reports to the Internal Revenue Service (IRS) by identifying the health needs of the communities in which they operate and the value of the non-compensated benefits they were providing to those communities (IOM, 2015). According to the statute's logic, the public reporting of needs and efforts to meet those needs will create greater accountability on the part of hospitals and health systems to address community-specific determinants of poor health, including social conditions. To date however, the potential for community benefit reporting has exceeded its accomplishments, with analyses of reports showing inconsistencies in the information reported to the IRS and limited national or local efforts to hold health systems accountable for the nature, extent, or efficacy of what is being reported (Rubin et al., 2015). In theory, increased and aligned expectations for health systems for how they are responding to the health needs of the communities they serve will result in more effective activities, including partnerships with other organizations responding to those needs. However, alignment between state and federal obligations varies as does the extent to which the approach taken to providing community benefits responds to the gap in social care. Efforts continue to align the IRS reports with local- and state-level health assessments, improvement plans, and policy (James, 2016; RTI International and RWJF, 2019).

Fragmented Financing for Dually Eligible Medicare and Medicaid Beneficiaries

A fourth challenge is the fragmented financing for dually eligible Medicare and Medicaid beneficiaries. If low-income populations have high social needs, older adults and people with disabilities with low incomes have some of the highest social needs. Not only do these "dual eligibles" have lives marked by considerable complexity of medical and social needs, but also those needs manifest themselves uniquely in each individual. For instance, a quadriplegic person in rural Oklahoma will have a very different set of needs and resources at his or her disposal than a frail older adult in a nursing home in San Diego. Addressing those needs in effective ways requires substantial commitment and flexibility on the part of care providers and the entities that determine coverage and payment decisions. Compared to Medicare enrollees, dual eligibles are more likely to have three or more chronic conditions and twice as likely to report fair or poor health and have a cognitive or mental impairment (Cubanski et al., 2015). Dual eligibles are one of the highest cost groups for Medicare and Medicaid expenditures (CBO, 2013).

The joint financing structure for dual eligibles has not yet provided the financing flexibility needed to care for this complex population. Medicaid and Medicare each have a list of covered services. A doctor being paid by Medicare must interact with a vendor paid by Medicaid to arrange for durable medical equipment. Investments by one payer, such as home health aides paid for by Medicaid, can result in the benefits—in this case reduced hospital admissions—accruing to the other. This dilemma is magnified with a service that is covered by neither payer, such as social care integration and services. Medicare has an incentive to cover the service only if the benefits accrue as a reduction in Medicare-covered services, yet if the integration of social care into the health care setting were to benefit any population it would be the one with the highest social and medical needs (i.e., the dual-eligible groups). Recognizing this, the federal government has made at least three different efforts to integrate financing for dual eligibles (CMS, 2018). The expectation is that a single stream of financing and one list of covered benefits would free health plans and the providers with whom they contract to increase their awareness of the social needs of these patients, assist them in meeting those needs, and align efforts with other providers. In a letter on April 24, 2019, CMS further encouraged the states promoting three models to integrate Medicare and Medicaid financing streams: (1) expanding the Medicare-Medicaid Financial Alignment Initiative, (2) integrating care through a managed fee-for-service model, and (3) encouraging state-specific models (CMS, 2019b).

Programs of All-Inclusive Care for the Elderly

The PACE Innovation Act of 2015 established integrated Medicaid and Medicare financing to integrated delivery systems for services to almost exclusively dual-eligible beneficiaries at high risk for nursing home admissions (CMS, 2017c). Through comprehensive primary care integrated into a day-program setting, the program has a demonstrated ability to delay or postpone nursing home admissions.

One study found that, compared with risk-adjusted populations in fee-for-service Medicare and Medicaid, PACE enrollees had fewer hospital admissions, more nursing home admissions, higher Medicaid costs (with the difference diminishing over time), no difference in Medicare costs, and lower mortality rates (Ghosh et al., 2014). Enrollment from 2007 to 2017 increased from 1.3 million nationwide to 4 million out of an estimated 9 million dual eligibles (CMS, 2017a).

Dual-Eligible Special Needs Programs

Dual-eligible special needs programs (D-SNP) seek to direct Medicare Advantage payments and Medicaid capitation payments to a single MCO responsible for administering both benefits. Whereas the 2018 budget agreement permanently authorized their status and estimated that 1.7 million potential beneficiaries reside in the 10 states that require their MCOs working with dual-eligible beneficiaries to become D-SNPs (Allen, 2018), no evaluations could be located by the committee. This perhaps is due to the varying nature of D-SNPs by state based on state Medicaid dual-eligible strategy and the joint accountability of D-DNP plans to Medicare and Medicaid.

In addition, the CHRONIC Care Act of 2018[4] makes explicit that care coordination and integration are central to the purpose of special needs plans (SNPs) as well as permanently authorizing SNPs and promoting home-based care with the goal of avoiding institutional care. As part of overall integration, the act provides three options for integrating long-term services and supports and behavioral health services by 2021, further encouraging integrating social care for those who are dually eligible. Finally, the act also requires the Medicare Payment Advisory Commission, in consultation with the Medicaid and Children's Health Insurance Program Payment and Access Commission, to conduct a study and report to Congress on the quality of D-SNPs. This strengthening and standardization of the D-SNPs is a step forward. However, financial alignment demonstrations seek to move further than what D-SNPs offer.

Financial Alignment Demonstrations

The ACA established an office in CMS to focus on the dual-eligible population and develop a set of financial alignment demonstrations, which resulted in joint agreements between CMS, a state Medicaid agency, and participating health plans on the categories of dual-eligible populations to be covered, covered services, payment rates, and accountabilities.

The financial alignment demonstrations allowed participating states to determine the amount of flexibility in how so called "value added" services are defined and financed. These services often were identified as social care for the dually eligible population. The states ranged in the amount of flexibility they allowed. For example, Minnesota defined "additional services" wherein MCOs were given full discretion to identify and pay for services that are not defined health care benefits and that these additional services must be made broadly available to all enrollees (Walsh, 2018b). Another example is California's use of "Care Plan Option" services (Walsh, 2018a). These services are optional services outside the defined benefits, which plans can purchase to enhance care, promote community living, and prevent costly and unnecessary hospitalization or prolonged institutional care. The intended outcome for these value-added services included filling in gaps in care, diverting enrollees from hospital or skilled nursing facility placements to promote community living, and improving physical health by addressing social needs (Soper, 2017).

---

[4] Title III of the Bipartisan Budget Act of 2018, Public Law 123, 115th Cong. (February 9, 2018).

The results are early and have been mixed. For example, the initial CMS evaluation in California noted no statistically significant savings under Medicare, a result that was attributed to a low initial enrollment and high variability of outcomes between participating MCOs. Ohio's evaluation, however, found lower monthly inpatient admissions and skilled nursing facility admissions, a lower probability of any long-stay nursing facility use, no effect on ER visits or all-cause 30-day readmission, and no effect on the probability of follow-up after inpatient mental health discharges. Washington demonstrated savings of $105.3 million for Medicare, and Illinois witnessed a 2.2 percent reduction in costs. Each of the evaluations documented challenges in financial sustainability, creativity in addressing social needs, and extension of the demonstration to accrue more data for analysis, given the overall promising results (CMS, 2019a).

Lack of Administrative Capacity for Social Service Providers

A final challenge to integrating social care into the health care setting is the administrative capacity of social service providers, which often are key to the delivery of social care. These providers are generally smaller organizations than their health care partners, and their funding usually is driven by grants, not service-related payments. They typically do not have systems in place for health care financing mechanisms. Historically, there has been little contracting or collaborating between the health care sector and social service providers.

In a medical model of health care, the workflow consists of generalists assessing needs, treating the patient if possible, and referring the patient to specialists for diagnosis, consultation, and possibly treatment. In an integrated social care model, social services providers represent another set of specialists and consultants with which the health care practice is collaborating. It is unlikely that the social service provider and the health care practice have established expectations for referral, consultation, feedback loops, reporting, and billing. Depending on the extent of the service integration desired and indicated, the integration of operational and management systems may be required. The potential for "medicalization" of social conditions (i.e., subsuming social services and public health under the health care delivery system) is of concern. This medicalization, if based on an overly formalized social care integration effort based on a medical model of diagnosis, assessment, referral, and treatment, may result in needless cost and complication, and may decrease the efficacy of the social care delivery (Lantz, 2018). This is a new dialogue, without the national standards provided by common definitions of condition and services, fee schedules, and reporting or contracting measures (CHCS, 2019). Coordination and communication between social service providers and health care providers in an integrated fashion may represent new administrative burdens and costs. It may create in social services providers a deeper cadre of skilled management professionals, or it may simply add administrative costs in the manner that has attracted concern and critique in health care (Papanicolas et al., 2018).

The committee did not research the costs involved to integrate social care into the delivery of health care as this exploration falls outside of the scope of this report.

FINDINGS

The challenges and opportunities in financing the integration of social care into health care fall into five categories: (1) definitions of health care, (2) payment reforms, (3) quality and accountability, (4) fragmented financing for dually eligible beneficiaries, and (5) a lack of administrative capacity for social care providers. What follows are the committee's findings based on the evidence.

- *Current health and social care spending*
  - Countries and states with a higher ratio of social to health care spending have better population health outcomes. Most of these countries have some form of global budgeting for health care expenses to limit the health care sector's growth.
  - A small portion of social spending is needed for the activities of social care integration in a health care setting: raising awareness, providing adjustments, assisting populations, and aligning activities.
- *Definition of health care and how it affects the inclusion of social care as part of health care*
  - The definitions in statute and in contracts of what constitutes health care have been driven in large part by the cultural history of medicine and have made it less likely that the activities of social care would be included in the health care setting. For example, social workers have been defined as mental health providers rather than more generally as health care providers.
  - Within existing statutory definitions of health care, state Medicaid programs and their contracted managed care plans and accountable providers are innovating with awareness, adjustment, assistance, and alignment activities to pay for social care in health care settings using state plan amendment authority and the waiver process. This activity is only beginning to scale in some states.

  - o There remains great variation among states in the level of social care activity; the guidance from the Centers for Medicare & Medicaid Services to states and from states to plans about permissible social care activities and benefits is limited.
  - o Rate-setting processes for health plans and providers can be influential in obtaining financing for the integration of social care in the health care setting; the key factors are the rates calculated, risk adjustment elements to those rates, performance incentives, and the definition of medical services and quality improvement activities in the calculation of medical loss ratios.
  - o Among the states with approved waivers there is much experimentation, with informal mechanisms for learning the results of the experimentation. Formal evaluations of these waiver activities typically are not timely and do not influence policy and practice.
  - o The Medicare Advantage plan bidding process insufficiently promotes competition on the basis of care coordination and high-quality care in the service of enrollees.
  - o Medicare's new supplemental benefits guidance to Medicare Advantage plans, made possible by the Creating High-Quality Results and Outcomes Necessary to Improve Chronic Care Act (CHRONIC Care Act), has created new opportunities to integrate social care into the health care of Medicare beneficiaries.
- *Incentives to integrate health care and social care*
  - o The prevailing model of health care provider payment—fee-for-service—does not encourage the integration of social care. The current shift to alternate payment models led by the Center for Medicare & Medicaid Innovation activities—particularly the shift to accountable care organizations—aligns incentives for the provision of social care.
  - o Just as state Medicaid programs are experimenting with different covered services definitions, they are innovating with new methods to pay providers, such as through accountable care organizations, in part to encourage more social care integration work. There is less such work taking place for commercial and Medicare populations. Furthermore, great variation among states exists in the types of population-based payment models (i.e., models in which a provider agrees to accept responsibility for the health of a group of patients in exchange for a set amount of money) that are being deployed, and, as with covered service definitions, states and, in some cases, their contracted health plans are not performing formal evaluation of these activities.

- *Quality and accountability*
  - o Definitions of health care services and conditions have historically provided insufficient clarity and guidance for the work of social care.
  - o Population outcome measures for accountable entities, or accountable care organizations, are numerous and highly variable among the states.
  - o The conclusions included in a previous National Academies of Sciences, Engineering, and Medicine report on adjusting Medicare payments for social risk factors (NASEM, 2017) have not been applied in Medicaid settings to payments or outcome measures.
  - o Even with good accountability measures, health plans and providers struggle to justify investments when returns are delayed and accrue to collaborators. The lack of continuous eligibility for Medicaid benefits exacerbates this problem, as does the long-term nature of the returns on investments in social care integration and on upstream investment in pediatric populations. Geographic exclusivity, which limits the number of providers operating within a region, makes it possible for partners to make longer-term investments, but this is not possible in populous settings.
  - o The Internal Revenue Service (IRS) community benefit standard is another opportunity to finance the integration of social care in health care settings. Experience has shown varying levels of engagement by health systems, little enforcement by the IRS, and varying levels of aligned attention from states and communities.
- *Financing care for patients with complex health and social needs*
  - o Patients enrolled in both Medicaid and Medicare have the highest social needs, but the division of their health care financing between state and federal agencies creates barriers to addressing those needs in a way that integrates social care.
  - o The Programs of All-Inclusive Care for the Elderly program enrolls a fraction of dual eligibles and has demonstrated mixed outcomes.
  - o No systematic evaluations exist for dual-eligible special needs programs (D-SNPs), in part because each is unique to the state in which it operates. The CHRONIC Care Act mandated the evaluation of D-SNPs, which may assist with standardization.
  - o The financial alignment demonstration for dual eligibles shows that while care innovation increases with alignment, administrative and financial challenges remain.

  - o Evaluations of the financial alignment demonstration have found savings in two states and improved health care use outcomes in additional states. The demonstration has been extended and expanded to accrue more of the data needed to evaluate its effectiveness.
- *Capacity building for social care providers*
  - o Social service agencies and health care organizations have historically not worked together. The systems of financing social services agencies and of financing health care organizations are different.
  - o Health systems may "medicalize" the integration of social care into health care. Health systems often use models of care requiring research, diagnostic codes, and technical specialization, which add cost and complexity, with the ultimate result being effects on population health that are neutral or negative.
  - o The administrative costs of social care providers could increase as a result of efforts to integrate social care into a health care setting based on a medical model for consultation and referral.

REFERENCES

AHA (American Hospital Association). 2018. *ICD-10-CM coding for social determinants of health.* http://www.ahacentraloffice.org/PDFS/2018PDFS/value-initiative-icd-10-code-sdoh-0418.pdf (accessed May 23, 2019).

Alderwick, H., C. M. Hood-Ronick, and L. Gottlieb. 2019. *Strategies for supporting Medicaid beneficiaries' social needs: A look at Oregon and California.* The Commonwealth Fund, May 6. https://www.commonwealthfund.org/publications/journal-article/2019/may/medicaid-beneficiaries-social-needs-oregon-california (accessed May 23, 2019).

Allen, K. 2018. *Companion Medicaid and Medicare Advantage dual-eligible special needs plans.* Health Management Associates blog. https://www.healthmanagement.com/blog/companion-medicaid-medicare-advantage-dual-eligible-special-needs-plans (accessed May 23, 2019).

Alley, D. E., C. N. Asomugha, P. H. Conway, and D. M. Sanghavi. 2016. Accountable health communities—Addressing social needs through Medicare and Medicaid. *New England Journal of Medicine* 374(1):8–11.

Arons, A., S. DeSilvey, C. Fichtenberg, and L. Gottlieb. 2018. Documenting social determinants of health-related clinical activities using standardized medical vocabularies. *Journal of the American Medical Informatics Association Open*. doi: 10.1093/jamiaopen/ooy051.

ASPE (U.S. Department of Health and Human Services' Office of the Assistant Secretary for Planning and Evaluation). 2018. *Report to Congress on the Medicaid health home state plan option.* https://www.medicaid.gov/state-resource-center/medicaid-state-technical-assistance/health-home-information-resource-center/downloads/medicaidhomehealthstateplanoptionrtc.pdf (accessed May 23, 2019).

Bachrach, D., J. Guyer, and A. Levin. 2016. Medicaid coverage of social interventions: A road map for states. *The Milbank Quarterly*, July 25. https://www.milbank.org/publications/medicaid-coverage-social-interventions-road-map-states (accessed August 28, 2019).

Bachrach, D., J. Guyer, S. Meier, J. Meerschaert, and S. Brandel. 2018. *Enabling sustainable investment in social interventions: A review of Medicaid managed care rate-setting tools*. The Commonwealth Fund, January 31. https://www.commonwealthfund.org/publications/fund-reports/2018/jan/enabling-sustainable-investment-social-interventions-review (accessed May 23, 2019).

Bodenheimer, T., R. A. Bereson, and P. Rudolf. 2007. The primary care–specialty income gap: Why it matters. *Annals of Internal Medicine* 146(4):301–306.

Bradley, E. H., and L. A. Taylor. 2013. *The American health care paradox: Why spending more is getting us less*. New York: Public Affairs.

Bradley, E. H., M. Canavan, E. Rogan, K. Talbert-Slagle, C. Ndumele, L. Taylor, and L. A. Curry. 2016. Variation in health outcomes: The role of spending on social services, public health, and health care, 2000–09. *Health Affairs (Millwood)* 35(5):760–768.

California Health Care Foundation. 2018. *Intended consequences: Modernizing Medi-Cal rate setting to improve health and manage costs*. https://www.chcf.org/publication/intended-consequences-modernizing-medi-cal-rate-setting-to-improve-health-and-manage-costs (accessed May 23, 2019).

CBO (Congressional Budget Office). 2013. *Dual-eligible beneficiaries of Medicare and Medicaid: Characteristics, health care spending, and evolving policies*. https://www.cbo.gov/sites/default/files/113th-congress-2013-2014/reports/44308dualeligibles2.pdf (accessed May 23, 2019).

Chaiyachati, K. H., D. T. Grande, and J. Aysola. 2016. Health systems tackling social determinants of health: Promises pitfalls, and opportunities of current policies. *American Journal of Managed Care* 22(11):e393–e394.

CHCS (Center for Health Care Strategies). 2017. *Quality measurement approaches of state Medicaid accountable care organization programs*. https://www.chcs.org/resource/quality-measurement-approaches-medicaid-accountable-care-organizations (accessed May 23, 2019).

CHCS. 2018. *Profiles*. https://www.chcs.org/resource/complex-care-innovation-action (accessed May 23, 2019).

CHCS. 2019. *Supporting social service and health care partnerships to address health-related social needs*. https://www.chcs.org/project/partnership-healthy-outcomes-bridging-community-based-human-services-health-care (accessed May 23, 2019).

CHCS/ACAP (Center for Health Care Strategies and Association for Community Affiliated Plans). 2018. *Addressing social determinants of health via Medicaid managed care contracts and Section 1115 demonstrations*. Webinar, December 11. https://www.chcs.org/resource/addressing-social-determinants-of-health-via-medicaid-managed-care-contracts-and-%C2%A7-1115-demonstrations (accessed May 23, 2019).

CMS (Centers for Medicare & Medicaid Services). 2015. *Application for a 1915(c) home and community-based waiver: Instructions, technical guide and review criteria*. https://www.medicaid.gov/medicaid-chip-program-information/by-topics/waivers/downloads/technical-guidance.pdf (accessed May 23, 2019).

CMS. 2016. *Chronic care management services*. https://www.cms.gov/outreach-and-education/medicare-learning-network-mln/mlnproducts/downloads/chroniccaremanagement.pdf (accessed May 23, 2019).

CMS. 2017a. 2017 *Programs of All-Inclusive Care for the Elderly (PACE) audit and enforcement report*. https://www.cms.gov/Medicare/Compliance-and-Audits/Part-C-and-Part-D-Compliance-and-Audits/Downloads/2017PACEAnnualReport.pdf (accessed May 22, 2019).

CMS. 2017b. *PACE Innovation Act*. https://www.cms.gov/Medicare-Medicaid-Coordination/Medicare-and-Medicaid-Coordination/Medicare-Medicaid-Coordination-Office/PACE/PACEInnovationAct.html (accessed March 20, 2019).

CMS. 2017c. *National health expenditures 2017 highlights*. https://www.cms.gov/research-statistics-data-and-systems/statistics-trends-and-reports/nationalhealthexpenddata/nationalhealthaccountshistorical.html (accessed March 20, 2019).

CMS. 2018. *Medicare–Medicaid Coordination Office*. https://www.cms.gov/Medicare-Medicaid-Coordination/Medicare-and-Medicaid-Coordination/Medicare-Medicaid-Coordination-Office/Downloads/FY-2018-Report-to-Congress.pdf (accessed March 20, 2019).

CMS. 2019a. *Evaluations*. https://www.cms.gov/Medicare-Medicaid-Coordination/Medicare-and-Medicaid-Coordination/Medicare-Medicaid-Coordination-Office/FinancialAlignmentInitiative/Evaluations.html (accessed May 23, 2019).

CMS. 2019b. *Three new opportunities to test innovative models of integrated care for individuals dually eligible for Medicaid and Medicare*. https://www.medicaid.gov/federal-policy-guidance/downloads/smd19002.pdf (accessed July 15, 2019)

Crumley, D., and P.-W. Marlise. 2018. *Addressing social determinants of health through Medicaid accountable care organizations*. Center for Health Care Strategies blog. https://www.chcs.org/addressing-social-determinants-health-medicaid-accountable-care-organizations (accessed May 23, 2019).

Cubanski, J., C. Swoope, G. Jacobson, G. Casillas, S. Griffin, and T. Neuman. 2015. *A primer on Medicare: Key facts about the Medicare program and the people it covers: What is the role of Medicare for dual-eligible beneficiaries?* Kaiser Family Foundation. https://www.kff.org/report-section/a-primer-on-medicare-what-is-the-role-of-medicare-for-dual-eligible-beneficiaries (accessed May 23, 2019).

Cuckler, G. A., A. M. Sisko, J. A. Poisal, S. P. Keehan, S. D. Smith, A. J. Madison, C. J. Wolfe, and J. C. Hardesty. 2018. National health expenditure projections, 2017–26: Despite uncertainty, fundamentals primarily drive spending growth. *Health Affairs* 37(3):482–492.

Flexner, A. 1910. *Medical education in the United States and Canada*. New York: Carnegie Foundation for the Advancement of Teaching.

GAO (U.S. Government Accountability Office). 2018. *Medicaid demonstrations: Evaluations yielded limited results, underscoring need for changes to federal policies and procedures*. GAO-18-220.

Gara, A. 2018. *Healthcare stocks plunge as Buffett, Bezos and Dimon team up to fight "tapeworm" costs on economy*. https://www.forbes.com/sites/antoinegara/2018/01/30/healthcare-stocks-plunge-as-buffett-bezos-and-dimon-team-up-to-fight-tapeworm-costs-on-economy (accessed February 5, 2019).

Ghosh, A., C. Orfield, and R. Schmitz. 2014. *Evaluating PACE: A review of the literature*. Mathematica Policy Research. https://aspe.hhs.gov/system/files/pdf/76976/PACELitRev.pdf (accessed May 23, 2019).

Gottlieb, L., R. Tobey, J. Cantor, D. Hessler, and N. E. Adler. 2016. Integrating social and medical data to improve population health: Opportunities and barriers. *Health Affairs (Millwood)* 35(11):2116–2123.

Gottlieb, L., N. Razon, and N. Aboelata. 2019. *How do safety net clinics pay for social care programs?* Social Interventions Research & Evaluation Network. https://sirenetwork.ucsf.edu/tools-resources/resources/how-do-safety-net-clinics-pay-social-care-programs (accessed May 23, 2019).

Improving Care for Medicare Beneficiaries with Chronic Conditions, Committee on Finance, U.S. Senate. 2015. *Statement of Mark E. Miller*. http://www.medpac.gov/docs/default-source/congressional-testimony/testimony-improving-care-for-beneficiaries-with-chronic-conditions-senate-finance-.pdf?sfvrsn=0 (accessed March 15, 2019).

IOM (Institute of Medicine). 2015. *Financing population health improvement: Workshop summary*. Washington, DC: The National Academies Press.

James, J. 2016. Nonprofit hospitals' community benefit requirements. *Health Affairs*, February 25. https://www.healthaffairs.org/do/10.1377/hpb20160225.954803/full/healthpolicybrief_153.pdf (accessed May 23, 2019).

Joynt, K. E., N. De Lew, S. H. SHeingold, P. H. Conway, K. Goodrich, and A. M. Epstein. 2017. Social risk factors and equity in medicare payment. *New England Journal of Medicine* 376(6):507–510.

Kaiser Family Foundation. 2018. Total Medicaid MCO enrollment. https://www.kff.org/other/state-indicator/total-medicaid-mco-enrollment (accessed March 28, 2019).

Kaiser Family Foundation. 2019. *10 things to know about Medicaid: Setting the facts straight*. https://www.kff.org/medicaid/issue-brief/10-things-to-know-about-medicaid-setting-the-facts-straight (accessed March 28, 2019).

Kissam, S. M., H. Beil, C. Cousart, L. M. Greenwald, and J. T. Lloyd. 2019. States encouraging value-based payment: Lessons from CMS's State Innovation Models initiative. *Milbank Quarterly*, April 7 [Epub ahead of print]. doi: 10.1111/1468-0009.12380.

KPMG. 2018. *Investing in social services as a core strategy for healthcare organizations: Developing the business case*. https://institutes.kpmg.us/content/dam/institutes/en/government/pdfs/2018/investing-social-services.pdf (accessed August 13, 2019).

Lantz, P. M. 2018. The medicalization of population health: Who will stay upstream? *Milbank Quarterly* 97(1):36–39.

Laugesen, M. J. 2017. *Fixing medical prices: How physicians are paid*. Cambridge, MA: Harvard University Press.

Lieberman, S. M., E. Trish, L. Adler, J. R. Antos, J. Bertko, and P. B. Ginsburg. 2018. *The case for reforming competitive bidding in Medicare Advantage*. USC–Brookings Schaeffer Initiative for Health Policy, May 10. https://www.brookings.edu/blog/usc-brookings-schaeffer-on-health-policy/2018/05/10/the-case-for-reforming-competitive-bidding-in-medicare-advantage (accessed May 23, 2019).

Long-Term Quality Alliance. 2018. *Medicare advantage's new supplemental benefit for 2019: Plan views and responses*. http://www.ltqa.org/wp-content/themes/ltqaMain/custom/images/LTQA-Report-on-MA-Flexible-Supplemental-Benefits-FINAL-11-9-18.pdf (accessed May 23, 2019).

Machledt, D. 2017. Addressing the social determinants of health through Medicaid managed care. *Issue Brief (Commonwealth Fund)* 1–9.

MassHealth, Commonwealth of Massachusetts. 2018. *MassHealth accountable care organizations*. https://massdocsdigitalmassgov.s3.amazonaws.com/s3fspublic/2018/MassHealth%2520ACO%2520One-Pager_0.pdf?HQAkdYxhMJTUv2ZGcn9IODj0Dm72uVJV (accessed May 23, 2019).

McWilliams, J. M., L. A. Hatfield, M. E. Chernew, B. E. Landon, and A. L. Schwartz. 2016. Early performance of accountable care organizations in Medicare. *New England Journal of Medicine* 374:2357–2366.

Meyer, H. 2012. The coming experiments in integrating and coordinating care for "dual eligibles." *Health Affairs (Millwood)* 31(6):1151–1155.

Miller, B. M., D. E. Moore, W. W. Stead, and J. R. Balser. 2010. Beyond Flexner: A new model for continuous learning in the health professions. *Academic Medicine* 85(2):266–272.

MN DHS (Minnesota Department of Human Services). 2018. Accounting for social risk factors in Minnesota health care program payments. https://www.leg.state.mn.us/docs/2016/mandated/160992.pdf (accessed May 23, 2019).

NASEM (National Academies of Sciences, Engineering, and Medicine). 2017. *Accounting for social risk factors in medicare payment*. Washington, DC: The National Academies Press.

NC DHHS (North Carolina Department of Health and Human Services). 2018. *Healthy Opportunities Pilots facts sheet.* https://files.nc.gov/ncdhhs/SDOH-HealthyOpptys-FactSheet-FINAL-20181114.pdf (accessed May 23, 2019).

Papanicolas, I., L. R. Woskie, and A. K. Jha. 2018. Health care spending in the United States and other high-income countries. *JAMA* 319(10):1024–1039.

Roberts, E. T., A. M. Zaslavsky, and J. M. McWilliams. 2018. The value-based payment modifier: Program outcomes and implications for disparities. *Annals of Internal Medicine* 168(4):255–265.

RTI International and RWJF (Robert Wood Johnson Foundation). 2019. *Community benefit insight: Promoting transparency to inspire action.* http://www.communitybenefitinsight.org (accessed May 23, 2019).

Rubin, D. B., S. R. Singh, and G. J. Young. 2015. Tax-exempt hospitals and community benefit: New directions in policy and practice. *Annual Review of Public Health* 36:545–557.

Rubin, J., J. Taylor, J. Krapels, A. Sutherland, M. Felician, J. L. Liu, L. M. Davis, and C. Rohr. 2016. *Are better health outcomes related to social expenditure?* Santa Monica, CA: RAND. https://www.rand.org/pubs/research_reports/RR1252.html (accessed May 23, 2019).

Schoen, C., M. M. Doty, S. R. Collins, and A. L. Holmgren. 2005. Insured but not protected: How many adults are underinsured? *Health Affairs (Millwood) Supplemental Web Exclusives* W5-289–W5-302.

Shrank, W. H., D. J. Keyser, and J. G. Lovelace. 2018. Redistributing investment in health and social services—The evolving role of managed care. *JAMA* 320(21):2197–2198.

Soper, M. H. 2017. *Providing value-added services for Medicare–Medicaid enrollees: Considerations for integrated health plans.* Center for Health Care Strategies technical assistance brief. January. https://www.chcs.org/media/PRIDE-Value-Added-Services_012617.pdf (accessed May 23, 2019).

Squires, D., and C. Anderson. 2015. U.S. healthcare from a global perspective: Spending, prices, and health in 13 countries. *Issue Brief, Commonwealth Fund* 15:1–15.

Stock, R., and B. Goldberg. 2017. *Health reform policy to practice: Oregon's path to a sustainable health system: A study in innovation.* San Diego, CA: Elsevier.

Stoesz, D. 2014. Evidence-based policy: Reorganizing social services through accountable care organizations and social impact bonds. *Research on Social Work Practice* 24(2):181–185.

Super, N., M. Kaschak, and E. Blair. 2018. *Health care and community-based organizations have finally begun partnering to integrate health and long-term care.* Health Affairs blog, February 2. https://www.healthaffairs.org/do/10.1377/hblog20180130.620899/full (accessed May 23, 2019).

Swartz, K., P. F. Short, D. R. Graefe, and N. Uberoi. 2015. Reducing Medicaid churning: Extending eligibility for twelve months or to end of calendar year is most effective. *Health Affairs (Millwood)* 34(7):1180–1187.

Taylor, L. A., and L. M. Nichols. 2018. Social determinants as public goods: A new approach to financing key investments in healthy communities. *Health Affairs* 37(8):1223–1230.

Torres, J. M., J. Lawlor, J. D. Colvin, M. R. Sills, J. L. Bettenhausen, A. Davidson, G. J. Cutler, M. Hall, and L. M. Gottlieb. 2017. ICD social codes: An underutilized resource for tracking social needs. *Medical Care* 55(9):810–816.

Urban Institute. 2017. *What is the "wrong pockets problem"?* https://pfs.urban.org/faq/what-wrong-pockets-problem (accessed May 23, 2019).

Walsh, E. G. 2018a. *Financial alignment initiative California Cal MediConnect: First evaluation report.* RTI International. https://innovation.cms.gov/files/reports/fai-ca-firstevalrpt.pdf (accessed May 23, 2019).

Walsh, E. G. 2018b. *Minnesota demonstration to align administrative functions for improvements in beneficiary experience: Second evaluation report*. RTI International. https://innovation.cms.gov/Files/reports/fai-mn-secondevalrpt.pdf (accessed May 23, 2019).

Wynne, B., and M. Horowitz. 2018. *With great power comes great responsibility: Medicare Advantage's newfound supplemental benefit flexibility*. The Point. The Commonwealth Fund blog, June 7. https://www.commonwealthfund.org/blog/2018/great-power-comes-great-responsibility-medicare-advantages-newfound-supplemental-benefit (accessed February 5, 2019).

6

Implementing Awareness, Adjustment, and Assistance Strategies in Health Care Delivery Settings: Challenges and Potential Solutions

The committee reviewed a range of approaches that health care sector stakeholders have used to improve social care in health care delivery settings. These approaches are likely to face implementation barriers. Therefore, this chapter discusses the implementation challenges associated with social risk documentation and interventions specific to health care delivery settings (awareness, adjustment, and assistance strategies). Though the committee recognizes the gaps in efficacy and effectiveness evidence about such strategies, it also recognizes that social care integration's impact—and the ability to test its impact—will be closely linked to the effectiveness of its implementation. The committee, therefore, drew on the peer-reviewed and gray literature and on expert testimony to identify potential challenges to health care delivery-based activities to identify and intervene on social risk factors.

This chapter's focus is on implementation barriers associated with *awareness*, *adjustment*, and *assistance* activities that can support social care integration. The committee does not address challenges to implementing *alignment* or *advocacy* approaches, but instead focuses this chapter on the challenges likely to be faced in implementing within-clinic activities, as these usually must be accomplished before alignment or advocacy can be undertaken. Challenges in alignment or advocacy approaches are also likely.

This overview is not intended to discourage health care systems from implementing social care programs, but rather to facilitate such integration by describing potential implementation pitfalls and highlighting strategies that have been used in some settings to avoid or overcome them. Tables throughout this chapter offer potential strategies to address these key implementation challenges. These strategies are described in greater detail in the section on Implementation Strategies to Overcome Challenges. Examples of health care providers seeking to overcome implementation barriers associated with social care integration can be found in many of the references cited here, including Adams et al. (2017), Burkhardt et al. (2012), Gold et al. (2018), Hamilton et al. (2013), Joshi et al. (2018), Knowles et al. (2018), and LaForge et al. (2018).

CHALLENGES TO INITIATING SOCIAL CARE INTEGRATION

Before social care can be integrated into health care settings, the challenges to initiating such integration must be addressed. These challenges may include, for example, obtaining leadership support and staff buy-in, including new voices from those with expertise in social care alongside traditional health care professionals, and resolving logistical and operational issues.

Health system leadership must buy in to social care integration and be willing to both innovate and prioritize social care integration (Boyce, 2014; Institute for Alternative Futures, 2012). Leadership support may be affected by a number of factors, including system-level challenges, such as limited resources in the face of rising costs of delivering care, regulatory and reporting requirements, and the need to adapt operations and provide ongoing training.

Providers and staff may be concerned that social care integration will involve additional tasks that will compete with limited resources (LaForge et al., 2018; Tong et al., 2018). As evidence to support the integration of social care into health care is nascent, providers may believe that integrating social care into health care may not be impactful enough to justify investing in such integration or may be hesitant to take on unproven approaches.

Support for initiating social care integration may be affected by the organizational culture among staff and leadership as it relates to social care in health care. Some staff may not consider addressing social needs to be part of their job or may think that social needs cannot be addressed from health care settings or may doubt that addressing these needs helps patients (Andermann, 2018; Tong et al., 2018).

Logistical challenges can also take substantial resources and time to address (Institute for Alternative Futures, 2012). Some of these challenges include

- *Goal setting*. Clinics must first establish goals for social care integration—for example, which patients to screen and how screening data will be used—with little empirical guidance. Goals should account for staff capacity, patient population characteristics, the availability of community resources, existing clinic resources and partnerships, known areas of community need, and current screening practices.
- *Strategy and structure*. A coordinated strategy for social care integration may involve planning for project management, staff engagement, testing and iterating integration, workflows, designating staff to oversee integration, communication, and working with external partners (Institute for Alternative Futures, 2012; Pescheny et al., 2018; Thomas-Henkel and Schulman, 2017).
- *Infrastructure*. Social care integration requires having enough clinic staff to conduct related tasks. If the integration will involve referrals to social service agencies, community partnerships for such referrals may need to be established, along with a maintenance plan (Boyce et al., 2014) and an evaluation plan. If electronic documentation of social risks is desired, the technology (e.g., the ability to document social needs) to support the effort must be put in place, and staff who will use this technology must be trained and given access to it. Payment structures must be identified, especially in under-resourced care settings, with a maintenance plan (Byhoff et al., 2017; Gunderson et al., 2018; Institute for Alternative Futures, 2012). Value propositions (such as improving quality measures or reducing total cost of care) also must be identified.

Workflow, staffing, and technological challenges—and the methods for addressing them—are discussed in greater detail later in this chapter. Table 6-1 provides a summary of common implementation barriers and potential strategies for initiating social care integration. Establishing payments for social care integration is covered in Chapter 5.

CHALLENGES TO DOCUMENTING AND RESPONDING TO SOCIAL NEEDS

Various potential challenges to documenting and responding to social needs are described here. Identifying social needs is a critical first step to the integration of these needs into health care. Some organizations may want to begin by simply documenting social needs; others will also want to develop systems to respond to these needs. The challenges to documenting and responding to these needs may differ across organizations

TABLE 6-1
Potential Strategies for Initiating Social Care Integration

Phase	Potential Challenges	Strategies to Address These Challenges
Initiating Social Care Integration	Leadership support	Obtain formal commitment from leaders
	Provider and staff buy-in	Identify and prepare champions
	Organizational culture	Engage staff in planning
	Logistics	Develop clear protocols
	Goals	Assess local needs and resources, identify barriers
	Strategy	Develop a formal implementation plan
	Structure	Revise professional roles and workflows
	Infrastructure	Adapt payments structures, technology, staffing, or partnerships

and health care settings. See Table 6-2 for a summary of challenges to documenting and identifying social needs and potential strategies to address these challenges.

Challenges to Documenting Social Needs

Logistical

The challenges to identifying and documenting patients' social needs may include identifying a target population, selecting screening tools, designing workflows, creating staffing plans, providing appropriate training, obtaining the needed technological tools, and making rollout plans. The questions that need to be answered include

- *Which patients?* Practices must decide which patients and which needs to screen for or how often screening should occur with little guidance or evidence (O'Gurek and Henke, 2018).
- *Which screening tool or tools?* Numerous social needs screening tools exist, but none has been validated to predict specific outcomes, and no standardization exists (O'Gurek and Henke, 2018). Practices must select a tool without guidance. No one tool will meet all of their needs (LaForge et al., 2018). Practices may want to screen for specific social needs if they have partnerships with certain local agencies or avoid others if they lack such partnerships. There is little guidance to suggest how to adapt existing

TABLE 6-2
Potential Strategies for Documenting and Identifying Social Needs

Phase	Potential Challenges		Strategies to Address These Challenges
Documenting Social Needs	Logistics	Which patients	Learn from early adopters, assess local needs and resources, obtain and use patient feedback, use an implementation advisor
		Which tool	Assess local needs and resources, obtain and use patient feedback
		Which workflow	Revise professional roles and workflows, conduct small tests of change
		When	Revise professional roles and workflows, purposely reexamine the implementation
		How to administer	Revise professional roles and workflows, use an implementation advisor
		Who will administer	Revise professional roles and workflows, create new clinical teams
		Planning for roll out	Conduct small tests of change, purposely reexamine the implementation
		Staffing	Revise professional roles, conduct ongoing training
		Use of technology	Promote adaptability, use quality monitoring
Identifying Social Needs	Provider and staff	Perceived lack of resources	Alter incentives
		Do not see the need	Share data with clinicians
		May not feel comfortable	Engage patients to increase demand
		Overburdened	Revise professional roles and workflows, create new clinical teams
		May not want to change	Identify and prepare clinical champions
	Patient	Not receptive	Involve patients in planning
		Unprepared on embarrassed	Prepare patients to be active participants
		Unmotivated to take action	Explore patient barriers to action, prepare patients to be active participants
		Screening type	Obtain and use patient feedback
		Clinical relationship	Develop patient-centered language to discuss screening efforts

tools to meet local needs, as is often desired; furthermore, such adaptation can create barriers to scale-up, as discussed below (Gold et al., 2017; LaForge et al., 2018). Practices choosing a screening tool might consider how the collected data will be used, which social needs can be addressed with local resources, which screening tool fits the clinic's workflows, and the needed granularity of social needs data (e.g., specific financial needs rather than general financial strain) (Gold et al., 2017, 2018; Jensen et al., 2015; Thomas-Henkel and Schulman, 2017).

- *Which workflows?* Practices must identify effective social needs screening workflows; ideally, these will integrate into existing workflows (Jensen et al., 2015; Joshi et al., 2018; Stehlik et al., 2017). When identifying workflows, consideration should be given to when the data will be used and to making sure that the data are entered in time. Overall, successful data collection may involve flexibility in where, how, and by whom data are collected. The optimization of these workflows also involves having adequate staff and time and the appropriate technological resources for the data collection.
    - *When will social needs screening occur?* Timing challenges include the difficulty and time-consuming nature of reaching some patients, ensuring accessibility of social needs information during practice visits, patients' ability to complete the screening quickly, and patient ability to enter data using tools such as Web portals (Jensen et al., 2015; Katz et al., 2008; Thomas et al., 2018).
    - *How will social needs screening be administered?* There is little evidence to indicate which data collection mode patients prefer (Gottlieb et al., 2015; LaForge et al., 2018). Paper forms may be difficult for some patients to complete (Beck et al., 2012; Craig and Calleja Lorenzo, 2014; Thomas et al., 2018). Staff-led screenings and real-time data entry may delay workflows (Gold et al., 2017, 2018). Using tablets and kiosks requires creating and maintaining electronic health record (EHR) connections and tracking and sterilizing the devices; technological glitches can prevent data capture (Jensen et al., 2015), and some clinics and staff may not have access to these technologies (Craig and Calleja Lorenzo, 2014).
- *How to staff for social needs screening?* Social care integration may involve hiring new staff, removing staff from other activities, or adding to existing workloads. Screening conducted by non-clinical staff (e.g., community health workers) may avoid burdening the clinical staff, but such staff must still be hired, paid, trained,

given EHR access, and supervised; furthermore, these professions have high burnout rates (Bonney and Chang, 2018; Gunderson et al., 2018; Joshi et al., 2018; Pescheny et al., 2018; Rogers et al., 2018). Staff with time to conduct social needs screening may not be those best suited for the task (Thomas-Henkel and Schulman, 2017). Volunteers may be able to conduct social needs screening, but they may not be able to maintain regular schedules, turnover may necessitate finding and training replacements, volunteers may need access to data entry tools to ensure consistent record keeping, and patients may be uncomfortable with volunteers (Pescheny et al., 2018).

- *How and when to provide training?* Training staff to conduct social needs screening requires conducting a needs assessment of the targeted learners, developing or identifying an appropriate curriculum, identifying appropriate educational methodologies, selecting and training the trainers, creating an evaluation plan, and allocating funding, time, and space for the training to occur.
- *Do the available technological tools support social needs screening?* Practices using paper-based screening for social risk factors will struggle to track social needs or related referrals. EHR documentation, though preferable, can pose its own challenges (Joshi et al., 2018). These include having the ability to set up or adapt EHR-based social needs documentation (Gold et al., 2017; Stehlik et al., 2017), ensuring that the EHR supports standardized, user-friendly documentation (Adams et al., 2017; Hripcsak et al., 2015; Pinto et al., 2016; Stehlik et al., 2017) and data exchange with clinical partners (Hripcsak et al., 2015; Jensen et al., 2015; Joshi et al., 2018; Stehlik et al., 2017), and coding for social needs and referrals without national standards for doing so (Adams et al., 2017; Gottlieb et al., 2014; Hewner et al., 2017; Lewis et al., 2016; Monsen et al., 2018).
- *How to "roll out" social needs screening?* The implementation of social needs workflows may falter if the change is applied to an entire organization all at once.

Provider and Staff Challenges to Identifying Social Needs

When implementing social needs screening, the challenges from staff may include discomfort with such screening in general or when no referral is feasible, doubt about why such screening is needed, a lack of time to conduct screening, a lack of training, and difficulty in overcoming previous habits.

Some staff may not think social needs screening is needed or useful (Colvin et al., 2016; Tong et al., 2018) or that it should be addressed by health care staff (Adams et al., 2017; Andermann, 2018; Gold et al., 2017; Nelson et al., 2015; Palacio et al., 2018; Thomas et al., 2018; Tong et al., 2018). Some may think that they know the patient's situation, question the need for standardized screening, prefer an individualized approach, feel that there is inadequate evidence of the impact of managing social care to justify the effort involved in such integration, or think that patients will not seek out social care resources even if referred (Nelson et al., 2015; Pescheny et al., 2018; Thomas et al., 2018). Some may struggle to change practice habits to include social needs screening (Andermann, 2018; Pescheny et al., 2018), and some may not screen universally, sometimes acting on biases and assumptions about whether a given patient should be screened. Some may lack the EHR expertise needed for screening documentation or find the EHR documentation tools difficult to use or inaccessible to certain staff (Gold et al., 2017). Some may feel too overworked to add social needs screening to their workload, and they may not want to add time to the visit, especially if social needs screening seems incongruous with the visit's primary purpose (Andermann, 2018; Joshi et al., 2018; Knowles et al., 2018; Palacio et al., 2018; Ridgeway et al., 2013; Thomas et al., 2018; Tong et al., 2018).

Staff may not want to screen for social needs if there are not resources to which they can refer patients to address those needs (Andermann, 2018; Olayiwola et al., 2018; Palacio et al., 2018; Pescheny et al., 2018; Purnell et al., 2018); this situation can cause burnout (Olayiwola et al., 2018; Tong et al., 2018). Staff may feel uncomfortable asking about social needs, overwhelmed by the need they encounter (Andermann, 2018), or apprehensive about their ability to address needs (Palacio et al., 2018; Pescheny et al., 2018; Purnell et al., 2018; Ridgeway et al., 2013). In addition, staff may not want to offend or disturb patients by asking about social needs (Beck et al., 2012; Gold et al., 2017; Hewner et al., 2017; Meredith et al., 2017; Saberi et al., 2017; Thomas-Henkel and Schulman, 2017) or make patients feel stigmatized (although anecdotal evidence suggests that this concern is often unwarranted) (Adams et al., 2017; Knowles et al., 2018). Finally, some staff may experience social needs themselves.[1]

Patient Challenges to Identifying Their Own Social Needs

Patients may or may not be receptive to social needs screening (Adams et al., 2017; Garg et al., 2007; Jaganath et al., 2018; Katz et al., 2008; Pinto et al., 2016; Quinn et al., 2018; Saxe-Custack et al., 2018). They may feel unprepared to discuss their needs (Katz et al., 2008), embarrassed to discuss their finances (Nguyen et al., 2018; Thomas et al., 2018), unmotivated to

[1] Personal communication, Robyn Gold, Rush University, April 18, 2019.

act on their needs, concerned about the legal ramifications of accessing social services (e.g., effect on immigration status), or generally concerned about stigmatization (Pescheny et al., 2018). However, staff should not assume that patients will resist such screening. Patient discomfort may depend on the specific needs (Thomas et al., 2018; Vest et al., 2017) or on their trust of clinic staff (Knowles et al., 2018). Some patients may prefer to disclose sensitive information to providers and staff with whom they share a racial/ethnic, social class, or cultural background, or those who at least demonstrate cultural humility and knowledge of structural determinants of health; this strengthens the argument for a more diverse and culturally competent workforce (Cooper et al., 2003; Murphy et al., 2018).

Challenges to Responding to Social Needs

Some challenges to responding to social needs are similar to those for social needs documentation, but some are unique, such as identifying referral resources, creating and maintaining partnerships with social service providers, and establishing needed data exchanges. Tables 6-3, 6-4, and 6-5 list common challenges to reviewing and responding to social needs and potential strategies to address these challenges.

Challenges to Reviewing Social Risk Data

To successfully integrate social care into health care, processes for reviewing, analyzing, and acting on patient-reported data and communicating results across care team members must be developed and tested

TABLE 6-3
Potential Strategies for Reviewing and Responding to Social Needs

Phase	Potential Challenges	Strategies to Address These Challenges
Reviewing Social Needs	Identify a process	Conduct small tests of change, promote adaptability
	Identify workflow	Engage staff in planning, revise professional role and workflows
	Lack incentives	Alter incentives, mandate change
	Retrieving and reviewing results	Conduct small tests of change
	Which needs require a response	Involve patients in planning, learn from early adopters, assess local needs and resources
	Data easy to find and interpret	Conduct small tests of change, use data experts

TABLE 6-4
Potential Strategies for Internal Referrals

Phase	Potential Challenges		Strategies to Address These Challenges
Internal Referrals	Logistics	Staffing and workflow	Revise professional roles and workflows, create new clinical teams, ensure adequate staffing
		Technology/clear documentation	Modify record systems, conduct ongoing training, provide ongoing consultation
	Staff	Role confusion	Revise professional roles, conduct ongoing training
		Lack of buy-in/ incentives	Identify and prepare champions, modify incentives, mandate change
	Patient	Patients may not accept support	Involve patients in planning, address patient provider trust
		Patient desire for support not established	Involve patients in planning

(Boyce et al., 2014; O'Gurek and Henke, 2018; Pescheny et al., 2018). Effective workflows and staffing for reviewing social needs data must be identified (Andermann, 2018), with little evidence on best practices. If social care referrals are not planned or feasible, the staff may lack incentives to review the documented needs (Gold et al., 2018).

Screening results must be easy to retrieve and review in the EHR (Gold et al., 2018; Jensen et al., 2015; Katz et al., 2008; Vest et al., 2017), but such functionality is not yet in all EHR systems. Care teams must know how to locate these data in the EHR, and the appropriate staff must have access to those data; they also may want guidance on which needs require a response and on the optimal timeframe for that response (Gold et al., 2018; Katz et al., 2008). If staff do not know how to find, interpret, and act on documented social needs data, their review of such data may be limited (Hewner et al., 2017).

Challenges to Responding to Social Needs Data

Broadly speaking, practices may respond to patients' social needs by adapting care plans to account for these needs or by referring patients "internally" to a clinic social worker or care navigator, to resources provided by the clinic (e.g., food, transportation, or legal services), or externally to local social service agencies. The practice must decide which approach or

TABLE 6-5
Potential Strategies for External Referrals

Phase	Potential Challenges		Strategies to Address These Challenges
External Referrals	Logistics	Workflow—no appointment made	Adapt workflows, conduct small tests of change
		Staff roles	Clearly define team roles
		Knowledge of resources	Conduct assessment of local needs and resources
	Staff	Knowledge of resources	Conduct assessment of local needs and resources, develop and distribute educational materials
	Patient	Already have access	Conduct assessment of local needs and resource, involve patients in planning
		Negative past experiences	Obtain and use patient feedback
		Not confident in navigating the system	Prepare patients to be active participants, develop and distribute educational materials
		Do not believe CBOs can help	Obtain and use patient feedback, develop and distribute educational materials
		May have already taken action	Obtain and use patient feedback
		May only be interested in a medical solution	Obtain and use patient feedback, develop and distribute educational materials
		Fear—stigma, loss of benefit, deportation	Involve patients in planning, obtain and use patient feedback
		Lack transportation	Involve patients in planning, link patients to existing resources, build organizational networks
		Lack time	Revise workflows, involve patients in planning
		Patients lost to follow up	Involve patients in planning, prepare patients to be active participants

continued

NOTE: CBO = community-based organization.

TABLE 6-5
Continued

Phase	Potential Challenges		Strategies to Address These Challenges
External Referrals	Technology	Closing the loop	Use data experts, change record systems, conduct small tests of change
		Data privacy	Use data experts, change record systems
		Lack of CBO infrastructure	Provide local technical assistance, capture and share local knowledge
		Other barriers to data exchange	Use data experts
		Cost for social service lists	Refine or innovate billing practices
		Clinic staff unaware of technology for referrals	Conduct educational meetings, provide ongoing consultation
		Staff may not be able to access tools	Provide ongoing consultation
		May lack mechanism for noting referral in patient record	Use data experts, provide ongoing consultation
	Partnership	Establishing partnerships	Build coalitions, establish formal agreements
		Barriers to creating and maintaining partnerships	Identify and prepare community champions
		CBO capacity	Adapt payments structures, technology, staffing, or partnerships
		Lack of partnership experience	Offer training to CBO leadership
		Training and implementation support needed	Conduct educational meetings, provide ongoing consultation
		Effective cross-sector workflow	Conduct small tests of change, promote adaptability
		Reimbursement challenges	Refine or innovate billing practices
		CBO financial instability	Partner to seek alternative sources of funding
		Lack of methods for demonstrating partnership impacts	Consult with data and evaluation experts

approaches works best for its setting, considering priorities, initiatives, and payment structures; staff resources; available community resources; existing partnerships; and the known areas of need in the community.

Health care organizations may also use social needs data to inform resource allocation, community or policy advocacy, risk stratification, or partnership building. For example, an organization could justify its need for resources to payers and policy makers by presenting collected social needs data. It could also use these data in partnership with insurers to inform the design, implementation, and evaluation of health insurer–directed social service programs, such as medically tailored meal delivery, transportation, and housing. Social needs data could be used to argue for hiring care managers or to offer group visits, special classes, transportation services, income supplements for food or housing, or other services. These data also could be used to help community-based organizations (CBOs) co-develop programs or coordinate referrals. However, staff may not understand these uses of social needs data.

Adapting care plans While some of the ways that care plans might be adapted to address reported social needs are fairly intuitive (e.g., a patient without stable housing should not be prescribed a refrigerated medication), little evidence yet exists to guide such adaptation. Decision support related to social needs might help, but evidence is lacking upon which such decision support could be built.

Internal referrals

- Logistical challenges. Internal social needs referrals require identifying effective workflows with little guidance, ensuring that staff are available when needed, and obtaining and sustaining funding for this activity (Gunderson et al., 2018). Practices may have limited EHR capacity for supporting internal referrals (Gold et al., 2017, 2018; O'Gurek and Henke, 2018); if the EHR does not support referral documentation, the clinic staff may use less trackable work-arounds such as telephone and faxes (Craig and Calleja Lorenzo, 2014). The staff designated to address social needs may not be experienced in EHR documentation or have EHR access (Craig and Calleja Lorenzo, 2014).
- Staff challenges. Staff may feel role confusion (Andermann, 2018), turf-related tensions, lack of buy-in, or reluctance to engage in social care management (Jani et al., 2012).

External referrals

- Logistical challenges. If practices wish to refer patients to local social service agencies, one potential challenge is establishing effective workflows. Referrals to CBOs differ from clinical referrals in that they rarely involve making appointments. Few organizations have demonstrated effective processes for CBOs confirming that they served the patient (Lohr et al., 2018). The University of California, Los Angeles, Alzheimer's and Dementia Care Program established formal partnerships with CBOs that include systemized referrals and electronic communication mechanisms (Tan et al., 2014). If the workflow involves a one-on-one discussion with patients, space and time are needed for such conversations. Practices must determine which staff are best suited to make external social care referrals (Thomas-Henkel and Schulman, 2017); a person in this role will need time to engage with the patient, knowledge of local CBOs, and the ability to use the EHR as needed. Practices must establish and update a list of community service resources, which ideally can be accessed through the EHR (Adams et al., 2017; Andermann, 2018; Gold et al., 2017; LaForge et al., 2018; O'Gurek and Henke, 2018; Thomas-Henkel and Schulman, 2017). Businesses have emerged in recent years to provide and maintain such lists, and these service locators may help practices refer patients to CBOs and communicate and share data with CBOs. Options are discussed in the 2019 Community Resource Referral Platform guide from SIREN, which presents a useful overview (Cartier et al., 2019). Affordability of the service locators can be a challenge.
- Staff challenges. Practice staff may not understand which individual CBOs are available, what they do and which patients they serve, or how the referral process works (Knowles, 2018).
- Patient challenges. Not all patients with identified social needs desire clinic intervention to address those needs (Gold et al., 2017, 2018; Pescheny et al., 2018; Tong et al., 2018). They may already access the needed service; be ineligible for certain services; feel discomfort engaging with clinic staff about non-clinical needs; have negative past experiences with such services; lack confidence in navigating such systems on their own; doubt that CBOs can help them; not be ready to take action to address a given need; fear stigmatization, loss to benefits, or deportation; or lack transportation or the time to access such services (Knowles et al., 2018; Pescheny et al., 2018). If the clinic plans to follow up on reported social needs via outreach, patients can be hard to reach (Knowles et al., 2018).

- Technological challenges. Many technological challenges to making and documenting referrals to CBOs exist. EHR functions for listing social service agencies and documenting referrals to such agencies are emerging, but have not been tested. When a patient is referred to a CBO, ideally the medical practice and CBO would be able to communicate about this referral in real time, but challenges to "closing the loop" (i.e., informing the health care entity that the patient accessed the services to which they were referred) remain (Bonney and Chang, 2018; Cartier et al., 2019; Lohr et al., 2018). Sending data through the Web requires practice staff to exit the EHR and re-enter data. Data safety and patient privacy must be addressed, and regional laws and organizational policies may pose challenges (Ridgeway et al., 2013). CBOs may resist responding to practices if different methods are needed for different practices. CBOs may not have the technological infrastructure needed to send information (Amarasingham et al., 2018), nor the staff resources and motivation to respond to the medical practice. The businesses offering tools for data exchange between CBOs and medical settings should address some of these challenges (Amarasingham et al., 2018; Bonney and Chang, 2018; Quinn et al., 2018; Thomas-Henkel and Schulman, 2017) (see Chapter 4 for more details). When social care referrals are documented, clinics may need to document these as distinct from clinical referrals since the rate of closed referrals can be a quality measure.
- Challenges to creating partnerships with community agencies: health system perspective. Partnerships between CBOs and health care entities are becoming increasingly common. These partnerships address a variety of care coordination and social care needs. Health care–community partnerships, though fundamental for making effective social care referrals, have inherent challenges (Bonney and Chang, 2018; Institute for Alternative Futures, 2012; Pescheny et al., 2018; Thomas-Henkel and Schulman, 2017; Valentijn et al., 2015). The CBO must have the capacity to serve referred clients or the ability to accommodate expanded demand (Garg et al., 2007; Pescheny et al., 2018; Tong et al., 2018). Building partnerships takes time and commitment, and a partnership agreement and governance structure are needed from the start to clarify expectations. Health care systems may cover a large geographic area and therefore need to develop partnerships with multiple local CBOs.
    - CBOs and medical practices may lack experience in cross-service partnership (Jani et al., 2012). Trust is essential, but establishing trust may be challenging due to structural

inequalities. Practices may not understand how their partnership affects the CBO or the CBO's ability to engage as desired. Both parties may need training and implementation support to adopt this change (Amarasingham et al., 2018; Kunkel et al., 2018; Thomas-Henkel and Schulman, 2017). Effective cross-sector workflows are hard to establish (Amarasingham et al., 2018).

- o CBOs' financing and technological systems differ from those of medical practices. Equitable reimbursement models may be difficult to establish (Amarasingham et al., 2018; Bonney and Chang, 2018; Griffin et al., 2018; Gunderson et al., 2018; Thomas-Henkel and Schulman, 2017), which may be exacerbated by local policies on reimbursement. CBOs funded by short-term grants may struggle to sustain partnerships (Amarasingham et al., 2018; Gunderson et al., 2018; Pescheny et al., 2018). Related payment challenges and strategies are discussed in Chapter 5.
- o There also are challenges to studying the impact of medical–CBO partnerships, including that it may not be feasible to share or analyze the needed data, effects on health outcomes may not manifest quickly, and CBOs may not maintain records that enable identifying clients referred from a given clinic. These factors can make it hard to sustain such partnerships (Amarasingham et al., 2018; Institute for Alternative Futures, 2012). It should be noted that the privacy protections contained in the Health Insurance Portability and Accountability Act of 1996 may allow for sharing of patient data between medical practices and CBOs.

- Challenges to creating partnerships with community agencies: CBO perspective. CBOs may find clinic partnerships difficult for some of the reasons given above. They may need to establish new organizational relationships, which are possibly made more difficult by power imbalances with better-resourced medical practices. They may lack the staff or staff competencies needed to support such partnerships. They may be unsure whether they will benefit from entering into such partnerships with medical practices directly or through businesses that help coordinate such efforts. For example, CBO-staffed social workers partnering with a clinic to provide biopsychosocial assessment and case management as part of the interprofessional team may offer an effective intervention, but unless the practice refers with enough volume and agrees to share clinical, usage, and cost data with the CBO, it is difficult to develop a business case for the partnership, and funding may not be renewed (American Society on Aging, 2019). Finally, even if they are willing to send data to medical practices regarding services provided to patients, CBOs may not have the technology needed for such data exchange.

Challenges in scaling up social care integration It can be useful to start social care integration in a single practice and then expand; however, future scaling much be considered from the start. Adaptations that facilitate integration in a single setting, such as a local adaptation of screening tools, can lead to future barriers to scaling up. It is highly preferable that the same screening and referral mechanism be used for all systems involved in the scale-up. If CBO referral making is to be expanded, the capacity of CBOs in all affected regions must be considered; a network may need to be created by hiring one of the resource locator businesses that support such development.

IMPLEMENTATION STRATEGIES TO OVERCOME CHALLENGES TO INTEGRATING SOCIAL CARE AND HEALTH CARE

Dissemination and implementation science defines "implementation strategies" as diverse approaches to supporting practice change in some settings and situations (Proctor et al., 2013). Some strategies that might support social care integration are discussed here. Strategies for addressing challenges to social care integration will vary by context. Most of the strategies listed below have effectively supported organizational changes in some practices, but almost none has been assessed specifically for supporting social care integration (Hamilton et al., 2013; O'Gurek and Henke, 2018).

Prepare to Implement Social Care Integration

Whether health care hopes to integrate with social care by documenting a single need or by screening for and acting on many needs, the efforts will be enhanced by communicating a clear and strong commitment from leadership to making this change, creating a formal implementation plan, and putting the needed infrastructure in place before implementation begins. This effort may involve information technology tools for social care documentation and review (Burkhardt et al., 2012; Craig and Calleja Lorenzo, 2014; Gold et al., 2017, 2018; Hewner et al., 2017; Thomas et al., 2018), and some EHR vendors now provide such tools. Medical practices should ensure access to interpreter services or translate the clinic's social needs screening tool, as appropriate, for the practice's patient population (Purnell et al., 2018). Practices should also ensure that their staffing is adequate to support intended activities and that funding structures to support integration are in place. The practices will need to decide which patients are targeted for social needs screening, which social needs screening tool will be used, which codes will be used to document social needs, and what actions will be taken to address those needs. Delivery system redesign and practice change efforts should use relationship-centered care principles in setting goals and priorities for social care integration (Beach et al., 2006). As discussed above, preparations for social care integration must consider how such efforts will be scaled up.

Implementation Strategies Targeting Clinical Staff

Many strategies may help address provider and staff integration challenges, including

- *Identify and support a clinical champion* to oversee and advocate for social care integration, and give the champion authority and time for implementation activities. Ideally, this person will be trusted by clinical staff and an experienced EHR user (Andermann, 2018; Gold et al., 2018).
- *Engage staff in the planning process* (Craig and Calleja Lorenzo, 2014; Gold et al., 2017; Pescheny et al., 2018). Create shared understanding about social care integration to develop buy-in; this may include defining the expectations of clinic staff and community partners.
- *Conduct staff training* to cover why the practice is screening for social needs, how the practice will use social needs data to improve patient health, how to conduct and respond to social needs screenings, and how to use EHR tools for social needs screening and referral-making (Andermann, 2018; Burkhardt et al., 2012; Craig and Calleja Lorenzo, 2014; Gold et al., 2018; Pescheny et al., 2018; Stehlik et al., 2017; Thomas-Henkel and Schulman, 2017). Ongoing training may be needed after the social care integration plan is put into place, especially if it is revised or if the information technology tools change, and onboarding staff will need to be trained (Gold et al., 2017). If CBO partners are involved, conduct a joint practice–CBO staff training.
- *Provide clear protocols for social needs screening*, including which patients to screen for which social needs at which visits (Andermann, 2018).
- Provide well-designed *workflows* for social needs screening, considering data entry methods, a review of social needs data, staff availability and training needs, escalation to other team members (e.g., from community health worker to social worker), and other

logistics (Andermann, 2018; Gold et al., 2017, 2018; Joshi et al., 2018).

- *Demonstrate the utility of systematic, EHR-documented social needs screening*. In several studies, practice staff said such screening helped them understand their patients' needs, which increased their acceptance of this practice. Such data can be used for advocacy, risk stratification, and other purposes (Gold et al., 2018; Hewner et al., 2017; LaForge et al., 2018; Palacio et al., 2018; Tong et al., 2018). Analyze social needs data, and share it with clinic staff (Palacio et al., 2018).

Implementation Strategies Targeting Patients

Several strategies have been developed to inform patients about social needs screening and its potential benefits and to increase the likelihood that they will be receptive to being screened. These include

- *Explain to the patient why the social needs screening is being conducted*—for example, because all new patients are being screened, and it can affect care planning—so as to avoid having the patient feeling singled out or stigmatized (Knowles et al., 2018).
- *Communicate with all patients* via a practice newsletter, posters in the waiting room, and patient portals, so patients know what to expect (Pescheny et al., 2018).
- *Use trusted staff to conduct screening*. Ensure that the person conducting social needs screening is someone whom patients trust (Thomas et al., 2018).
- *Activate patients to participate in decision making* related to their care. Consider helping patients increase their self-efficacy so that they feel able to follow up on referrals to community resources (Andermann, 2018).

Implementation Strategies Targeting Clinic Workflows and Processes

The strategies described below are aimed at improving clinic workflow and processes:

- *Start small*, for example, by screening patients seen by one team or provider—or focusing on one screening question—on one day. Small tests of change can accelerate the adoption of social care integration workflows. Test and hone clinic social needs processes on a small scale, address problems, and then scale up. Use quality improvement techniques, such as plan-do-study-act cycles, to test and improve social needs processes and workflows. This approach in screening has been effective at supporting the adoption of social determinants into clinic workflows and health processes (Burkhardt et al., 2012; Pescheny et al., 2018).

- *Provide feedback data* to show medical practice staff and leadership on progress in implementing social care integration (Pescheny et al., 2018). This strategy will be necessary—but not sufficient on its own—to support this integration. Check screening rates data often to inform workflow adaptations, and check in with high and low performers (Adams et al., 2017; Andermann, 2018; Burkhardt et al., 2012; Katz et al., 2008; Knowles et al., 2018; Pescheny et al., 2018). Be sure to establish whether screened patients desire clinic-led social care intervention before taking action to provide such support (Gold et al., 2018; Pescheny et al., 2018).

Implementation Strategies Targeting Community Partners

Strategies that may help integration challenges experienced by CBOs are listed below.

- *Engage community stakeholders and partners* from the start, including public health agencies and county or city counterparts who lead other social sector agencies, including in housing, food, transportation, and education; identify common ground and goals (Bonney and Chang, 2018; Joshi et al., 2018; Thomas-Henkel and Schulman, 2017; Udow-Phillips et al., 2018).
- *Start small*, to address problems before expanding, and be realistic about the time needed (Pescheny et al., 2018; Udow-Phillips et al., 2018).
- *Train all partners* in social care integration and about how the partnership will work (Pescheny et al., 2018).
- *Build trust* by mutually setting clear goals and expectations at the start; by having staff from all partner organizations meet in person before implementation begins; by enabling regular, bidirectional communication, feedback, and collaborative problem-solving; by using bottom-up approaches to alignment and partnership; and by being willing to revise how the partnership works (Joshi et al., 2018; Pescheny et al., 2018; Udow-Phillips et al., 2018; Valentijn et al., 2015).
- *Monitor partnership activities regularly* to ensure that needed revisions are identified, goals are met, and no partner's capacity is overtaxed (Bonney and Chang, 2018).

- *Establish a governance structure* that describes leadership roles, which patients will be served, training requirements, financing and business processes, methods for measuring success, and legal aspects (Bonney and Chang, 2018; Pescheny et al., 2018; Udow-Phillips et al., 2018). Create a partnership agreement.
- *Establish the infrastructure needed for partnership activities*, including staffing, start-up and maintenance funding, a monitoring and improvement plan, and data sharing (ideally through "closing the loop" between partners serving the same patient) (Bonney and Chang, 2018).
- *Consider different partnership structures*, such as partnering with a single CBO that can link patients to an array of services, such as an aging and disability resource center or a medical–legal partnership (Hyatt Thorpe et al., 2017; Klein et al., 2013; Martinez et al., 2017; Pettignano et al., 2012; Regenstein et al., 2018; Salter et al., 2018; Sandel et al., 2010; Sege et al., 2015; Williamson et al., 2018). Alternately, join or create a community-wide spoke-and-hub or pathways model, wherein patients are connected to many services through multiple entry points (AHRQ, 2016; Bonney and Chang, 2018; Hostetter and Klein, 2017).
- *Work with partnering agencies and organizations to identify funding structures that support social care integration*; for example, some payers may require social needs screening and referrals, such as accountable care organizations (Amarasingham et al., 2018; Andermann, 2018; Bachrach et al., 2014, 2018; Crumley and Marlise, 2018). These structures are discussed in detail in Chapter 5.
- *Share data with CBO partners*, if possible in a way that is useful to the CBO.

REFERENCES

Adams, E., D. Hargunani, L. Hoffmann, G. Blaschke, J. Helm, and A. Koehler. 2017. Screening for food insecurity in pediatric primary care: A clinic's positive implementation experiences. *Journal of Health Care for the Poor and Underserved* 28(1):24–29.

AHRQ (Agency for Healthcare Research and Quality). 2016. *Pathways Community HUB Manual: A guide to identify and address risk factors, reduce costs, and improve outcomes.* https://innovations.ahrq.gov/sites/default/files/Guides/CommunityHubManual.pdf (accessed May 24, 2019).

Amarasingham, R., B. Kapoor, A. Karam, N. Nguyen, and B. Xie. 2018. Using community partnerships to integrate health and social services for high-need, high-cost patients. *Issue Brief (The Commonwealth Fund)* 2018:1–11.

American Society on Aging. 2019. *Aging and Disability Business Institute.* https://www.asaging.org/aging-and-disability-business-institute-0 (accessed April 9, 2019).

Andermann, A. 2018. Screening for social determinants of health in clinical care: Moving from the margins to the mainstream. *Public Health Reviews* 39:19.

Bachrach, D., H. Pfister, K. Wallis, and M. Lipson. 2014. *Addressing patients' social needs: An emerging business case for provider investment.* The Commonwealth Fund. https://www.commonwealthfund.org/sites/default/files/documents/___media_files_publications_fund_report_2014_may_1749_bachrach_addressing_patients_social_needs_v2.pdf (accessed May 24, 2019).

Bachrach, D., J. Guyer, S. Meier, J. Meerschaert, and S. Brandel. 2018. *Enabling sustainable investment in social interventions: A review of Medicaid managed care rate-setting tools.* The Commonwealth Fund. https://www.commonwealthfund.org/publications/fund-reports/2018/jan/enabling-sustainable-investment-social-interventions-review (accessed May 24, 2019).

Beach, M. C., T. Inui, and the Relationship-Centered Care Research Network. 2006. Relationship-centered care. A constructive reframing. *Journal of General Internal Medicine* 21(Suppl 1):S3–S8.

Beck, A. F., M. D. Klein, and R. S. Kahn. 2012. Identifying social risk via a clinical social history embedded in the electronic health record. *Clinical Pediatrics* 51(10):972–977.

Bonney, J., and D. I. Chang. 2018. *Community care coordination systems: Connecting patients to community services.* Nemours Children's Health System. https://www.academyhealth.org/sites/default/files/community_care_coordination_systems_may2018.pdf (accessed May 24, 2019).

Boyce, M. B., J. P. Browne, and J. Greenhalgh. 2014. The experiences of professionals with using information from patient-reported outcome measures to improve the quality of healthcare: A systematic review of qualitative research. *BMJ Quality & Safety* 23(6):508–518.

Burkhardt, M. C., A. F. Beck, P. H. Conway, R. S. Kahn, and M. D. Klein. 2012. Enhancing accurate identification of food insecurity using quality-improvement techniques. *Pediatrics* 129(2):e504–e510.

Byhoff, E., K. M. Freund, and A. Garg. 2017. Accelerating the implementation of social determinants of health interventions in internal medicine. *Journal of General Internal Medicine* 33(2):223–225.

Cartier, Y., C. Fichtenberg, and L. Gottlieb. 2019. *Community resource referral platforms: A guide for health care organizations.* Social Interventions Research & Evaluation Network. https://sirenetwork.ucsf.edu/sites/sirenetwork.ucsf.edu/files/wysiwyg/Community-Resource-Referral-Platforms-Guide.pdf (accessed May 24, 2019).

Colvin, J. D., J. L. Bettenhausen, K. D. Anderson-Carpenter, V. Collie-Akers, and P. J. Chung. 2016. Caregiver opinion of in-hospital screening for unmet social needs by pediatric residents. *Academic Pediatrics* 16(2):161–167.

Cooper, L. A, D. L. Roter, R. L. Johnson, D. E. Ford, D. M. Steinwachs, and N. R. Power. 2003. Patient-centered communication, ratings of care, and concordance of patient and physician race. *Annals of Internal Medicine* 139:907–915.

Craig, S. L., and M. V. Calleja Lorenzo. 2014. Can information and communication technologies support patient engagement? A review of opportunities and challenges in health social work. *Social Work in Health Care* 53(9):845–864.

Crumley, D., and P.-W. Marlise. 2018. *Addressing social determinants of health through Medicaid accountable care organizations.* Center for Health Care Strategies blog. https://www.chcs.org/addressing-social-determinants-health-medicaid-accountable-care-organizations (accessed May 24, 2019).

Garg, A., A. M. Butz, P. H. Dworkin, R. A. Lewis, R. E. Thompson, and J. R. Serwint. 2007. Improving the management of family psychosocial problems at low-income children's well-child care visits: The We Care project. *Pediatrics* 120(3):547–558.

Gold, R., E. Cottrell, A. Bunce, M. Middendorf, C. Hollombe, S. Cowburn, P. Mahr, and G. Melgar. 2017. Developing electronic health record (EHR) strategies related to health center patients' social determinants of health. *Journal of American Board of Family Medicine* 30(4):428–447.

Gold, R., A. Bruce, S. Cowburn, K. Dambrun, M. Dearing, M. Middendorf, N. Mossman, C. Hollombe, P. Mahr, G. Melgar, J. Davis, L. Gottlieb, and E. Cotrell. 2018. Adoption of social determinants of health EHR tools by community health centers. *Annals of Family Medicine* 16(5):399–407.

Gottlieb, L., D. Hessler, D. Long, A. Amaya, and N. Adler. 2014. A randomized trial on screening for social determinants of health: The iScreen study. *Pediatrics* 134(6):e1611–e1618.

Gottlieb, L. M., K. J. Tirozzi, R. Manchanda, A. R. Burns, and M. T. Sandel. 2015. Moving electronic medical records upstream: Incorporating social determinants of health. *American Journal of Preventive Medicine* 48(2):215–218.

Griffin, K., C. Nelson, L. Realmuto, and L. Weiss. 2018. *Partnerships between New York City health care institutions and community-based organizations.* Greater New York Hospital Assocation and The New York Academy of Medicine. https://nyam.org/media/filer_public/9f/5b/9f5b33a3-0795-4a1a-9b90-fa999e9ddf8e/hco_cbo_partnerships_digital.pdf (accessed May 24, 2019).

Gunderson, J. M., M. L. Wieland, O. Quirindongo-Cedeno, G. B. Asiedu, J. L. Ridgeway, M. W. O'Brien, T. M. Nelson, R. Buzard, C. Campbell, and J. W. Njeru. 2018. Community health workers as an extension of care coordination in primary care: A community-based cosupervisory model. *Journal of Ambulatory Care Management* 41(4):333–340.

Hamilton, A. B., A. N. Cohen, D. L. Glover, F. Whelan, E. Chemerinski, K. P. McNagny, D. Mullins, C. Reist, M. Schubert, and A. S. Young. 2013. Implementation of evidence based employment services in specialty mental health. *Health Services Research* 48(6 Pt 2):2224–2244.

Hewner, S., S. Casucci, S. Sullivan, F. Mistretta, Y. Xue, B. Johnson, R. Pratt, L. Lin, and C. Fox. 2017. Integrating social determinants of health into primary care clinical and informational workflow during care transitions. *eGEMS* 5(2):2.

Hostetter, M., and S. Klein. 2017. *In focus: Creating pathways and partnerships to address patients' social needs.* The Commonwealth Fund. June 21. https://www.commonwealthfund.org/publications/newsletter-article/2017/jun/focus-creating-pathways-and-partnerships-address-patients (accessed May 24, 2019).

Hripcsak, G., C. B. Forrest, P. F. Brennan, and W. W. Stead. 2015. Informatics to support the IOM social and behavioral domains and measures. *Journal of American Medical Informatics Association* 22(4):921–924.

Hyatt Thorpe, J., L. Cartwright-Smith, E. Gray, and M. Mongeon. 2017. *Information sharing in medical–legal partnerships: Foundational concepts and resources.* National Center for Medical Legal Partnership at the George Washington University. https://medical-legalpartnership.org/wp-content/uploads/2017/07/Information-Sharing-in-MLPs.pdf (accessed May 24, 2019).

Institute for Alternative Futures. 2012. *Community health centers: Leveraging the social determinants of health.* Alexandria, VA: Institute for Alternative Futures. http://www.altfutures.org/wp-content/uploads/2016/04/2012_Report_Community-Health-Centers-Leveraging-the-Social-Determinants-of-Health.pdf (accessed May 24, 2019).

Jaganath, D., K. Johnson, M. M. Tschudy, K. Topel, B. Stackhouse, and B. S. Solomon. 2018. Desirability of clinic-based financial services in urban pediatric primary care. *Journal of Pediatrics* 202:285–290.

Jani, J. S., C. Tice, and R. Wiseman. 2012. Assessing an interdisciplinary health care model: The Governor's Wellmobile Program. *Social Work in Health Care* 51(5):441–456.

Jensen, R. E., N. E. Rothrock, E. M. DeWitt, B. Spiegel, C. A. Tucker, H. M. Crane, C. B. Forrest, D. L. Patrick, R. Fredericksen, L. M. Shulman, D. Cella, and P. K. Crane. 2015. The role of technical advances in the adoption and integration of patient-reported outcomes in clinical care. *Medical Care* 53(2):153–159.

Joshi, K., S. Smith, S. D. Bolen, A. Obsborne, M. Benko, and E. Trapl. 2018. Implementing a produce prescription program for hypertensive patients in safety net clinics. *Health Promotion and Practice* 20(1):94–104.

Katz, K. S., S. M. Blake, R. A. Milligan, P. W. Sharps, D. White, B., M. F. Rodan, M. Rossi, and K. B. Murray. 2008. The design, implementation and acceptability of an integrated intervention to address multiple behavioral and psychosocial risk factors among pregnant African American women. *BMC Pregnancy and Childbirth* 8(1):22.

Klein, M. D., A. F. Beck, A. W. Henize, D. S. Parrish, E. E. Fink, and R. S. Kahn. 2013. Doctors and lawyers collaborating to help children: Outcomes from a successful partnership between professions. *Journal of Health Care for the Poor & Underserved* 24(3):1063–1073.

Knowles, M., S. Khan, D. Palakshappa, R. Cahill, E. Kruger, B. Poserina, G., B. Koch, and M. Chilton. 2018. Successes, challenges, and considerations for integrating referral into food insecurity screening in pediatric settings. *Journal of Health Care for the Poor and Underserved* 29(1):181–191.

Kunkel, S. R., A. Lackmeyer, J. K. Straker, and T. L. Wilson. 2018. *Community-based organizations and health care contracting: Building & strengthening partnerships.* Scripps Gerontology Center research brief. https://sc.lib.miamioh.edu/bitstream/handle/2374.MIA/6280/Kunkel-Community-Based-Organizations-and-Health-Care-Contracting.pdf (accessed May 24, 2019).

LaForge, K., R. Gold, E. Cottrell, A. E. Bunce, M. Proser, C. Hollombe, K. Dambrun, D. J. Cohen, and K. D. Clark. 2018. How 6 organizations developed tools and processes for social determinants of health screening in primary care: An overview. *Journal of Ambulatory Care Management* 41(1):2–14.

Lewis, J. H., K. Whelihan, I. Navarro, and K. R. Boyle. 2016. Community health center provider ability to identify, treat and account for the social determinants of health: A card study. *BMC Family Practice* 17:121.

Lohr, A. M., M. Ingram, A. V. Nunez, K. M. Reinschmidt, and S. C. Carvajal. 2018. Community–clinical linkages with community health workers in the United States: A scoping review. *Health Promotion Practice* 19(3):349–360.

Martinez, O., J. Boles, L.-M. Munoz, E. C. Levine, C. Ayamele, R. Eisenberg, J. Manusov, and J. Draine. 2017. Bridging health disparity gaps through the use of medical legal partnerships in patient care: A systematic review. *Journal of Law, Medicine & Ethics* 45(2):260–273.

Meredith, L. S., G. Azhar, A. Okunogbe, I. A. Canelo, J. E. Darling, A. E. Street, and E. M. Yano. 2017. Primary care providers with more experience and stronger self-efficacy beliefs regarding women veterans screen more frequently for interpersonal violence. *Women's Health Issues* 27(5):586–591.

Monsen, K. A., J. M. Rudenick, N. Kapinos, K. Warmbold, S. K. McMahon, and E. N. Schorr. 2018. Documentation of social determinants in electronic health records with and without standardized terminologies: A comparative study. *Proceedings of Singapore Healthcare* 28(1):39–47.

Nelson, E. C., E. Eftimovska, C. Lind, A. Hager, J. H. Wasson, and S. Linblad. 2015. Patient reported outcome measures in practice. *BMJ* 350:g7818.

Nguyen, O. K., R. T. Higashi, A. N. Makam, J. C. Mijares, and S. C. Lee. 2018. The influence of financial strain on health decision-making. *Journal of General Internal Medicine* 33(4):406–408.

O'Gurek, D. T., and C. Henke. 2018. A practical approach to screening for social determinants of health. *Family Practice Management* 25(3):7–12.

Olayiwola, J. N., R. Willard-Grace, K. Dubé, D. Hessler, R. Shunk, K. Grumbach, and L. Gottlieb. 2018. Higher perceived clinic capacity to address patients' social needs associated with lower burnout in primary care providers. *Journal of Health Care for the Poor and Underserved* 29(1):415–429.

Palacio, A., D. Seo, H. Medina, V. Singh, M. Suarez, and L. Tamariz. 2018. Provider perspectives on the collection of social determinants of health. *Population Health Management* 21(6):501–508.

Pescheny, J. V., Y. Pappas, and G. Randhawa. 2018. Facilitators and barriers of implementing and delivering social prescribing services: A systematic review. *BMC Health Services Research* 18(1):86.

Pettignano, R., S. B. Caley, and S. McLaren. 2012. The health law partnership: Adding a lawyer to the health care team reduces system costs and improves provider satisfaction. *Journal of Public Health Management & Practice* 18(4):E1–E3.

Pinto, A. D., G. Glattstein-Young, A. Mohamed, G. Bloch, F. H. Leung, and R. H. Glazier. 2016. Building a foundation to reduce health inequities: Routine collection of sociodemographic data in primary care. *Journal of the American Board of Family Medicine* 29(3):348–355.

Proctor, E. K., B. J. Powell, and J. C. McMillen. 2013. Implementation strategies: Recommendations for specifying and reporting. *Implementation Science* 8:139.

Purnell, T. S., J. Kimbrough Marshall, I. Olorundare, R. W. Stewart, S. Sisson, B. Gibbs, L. S. Feldman, A. Bertram, A. R. Green, and L. A. Cooper. 2018. Provider perceptions of the organization's cultural competence climate and their skills and behaviors targeting patient-centered care for socially at-risk populations. *Journal of Health Care for the Poor and Underserved* 29(1):481–496.

Quinn, C., K. Johnson, C. Raney, J. Baker, K. Topel, M. M. Tschudy, D. Jaganath, and B. S. Solomon. 2018. "In the clinic they know us": Preferences for clinic-based financial and employment services in urban pediatric primary care. *Academic Pediatrics* 18(8):912–919.

Regenstein, M., J. Trott, A. Williamson, and J. Theiss. 2018. Addressing social determinants of health through medical–legal partnerships. *Health Affairs (Millwood)* 37(3):378–385.

Ridgeway, J. L., T. J. Beebe, C. G. Chute, D. T. Eton, L. A. Hart, M. H. Frost, D. Jensen, V. M. Montori, J. G. Smith, S. A. Smith, A. D. Tan, K. J. Yost, J. Y. Ziegenfuss, and J. A. Sloan. 2013. A brief patient-reported outcomes quality of life (PROQOL) instrument to improve patient care. *PLOS Medicine* 10(11):PMC3825652.

Rogers, E. A., S. Turcotte Manser, J. Cleary, A. M. Joseph, E. M. Harwood, and K. T. Call. 2018. Integrating community health workers into medical homes. *Annals of Family Medicine* 16(1):14–20.

Saberi, E., N. Eather, S. Pascoe, M.-L. McFadzean, F. Doran, and M. Hutchinson. 2017. Ready, willing and able? A survey of clinicians' perceptions about domestic violence screening in a regional hospital emergency department. *Australasian Emergency Nursing Journal* 20(2):82–86.

Salter, A. S., G. T. Anderson, J. Gettinger, and S. Stigleman. 2018. Medical–legal partnership in western North Carolina. *North Carolina Medical Journal* 79(4):259–260.

Sandel, M., M. Hansen, R. Kahn, E. Lawton, E. Paul, V. Parker, S. Morton, and B. Zuckerman. 2010. Medical–legal partnerships: Transforming primary care by addressing the legal needs of vulnerable populations. *Health Affairs (Millwood)* 29(9):1697–1705.

Saxe-Custack, A., H. C. Lofton, M. Hanna-Attisha, C. Victor, G. Reyes, T. Ceja, and J. LaChance. 2018. Caregiver perceptions of a fruit and vegetable prescription programme for low-income paediatric patients. *Public Health Nutrition* 21(13):2497–2506.

Sege, R., G. Preer, S. J. Morton, H. Cabral, O. Morakinyo, V. Lee, C. Abreu, E. De Vos, and M. Kaplan-Sanoff. 2015. Medical–legal strategies to improve infant health care: A randomized trial. *Pediatrics* 136(1):97–106.

Stehlik, J., C. Rodriguez-Correa, J. A. Spertus, J. Biber, J. Nativi-Nicolau, S. Zickmund, B. A. Steinberg, D. C. Peritz, A. Walker, J. Hess, S. G. Drakos, A. G. Kfoury, J. C. Fang, C. H. Selzman, and R. Hess. 2017. Implementation of real-time assessment of patient-reported outcomes in a heart failure clinic: A feasibility study. *Journal of Cardiac Failure* 23(11):813–816.

Tan, Z. S., L. Jennings, and D. Reuben. 2014. Coordinated care management for dementia in a large academic health system. *Health Affairs (Millwood)* 33(4):619–625.

Thomas, B., S. Fitzpatrick, S. Sidani, and E. Gucciardi. 2018. Developing and implementing a food insecurity screening initiative for adult patients living with type 2 diabetes. *Canadian Journal of Diabetes* 42(3):257–262.

Thomas-Henkel, C., and M. Schulman. 2017. *Screening for social determinants of health in populations with complex needs: Implementation considerations.* Center for Health Care Strategies. https://www.chcs.org/media/SDOH-Complex-Care-Screening-Brief-102617.pdf (accessed May 24, 2019).

Tong, S. T., W. R. Liaw, P. Lail Kashiri, J. Pecsok, J. Rozman, A. Bazemore, and A. H. Kirst. 2018. Clinician experiences with screening for social needs in primary care. *Journal of the American Board of Family Medicine* 31(3):351–363.

Udow-Phillips, M., K. O'Grady, and P. Meadows. 2018. *Nine lessons for leaders of health and human services integration initiatives (and for the grantmakers that want them to succeed).* Health Affairs blog. https://www.healthaffairs.org/do/10.1377/hblog20180709.359520/full (accessed May 24, 2019).

Valentijn, P. P., D. Ruwaard, H. J. Vrijhoef, A. de Bont, R. Y. Arends, and M. A. Bruijnzeels. 2015. Collaboration processes and perceived effectiveness of integrated care projects in primary care: A longitudinal mixed-methods study. *BMC Health Services Research* 15:463.

Vest, J. R., S. J. Grannis, D. P. Haut, P. K. Halverson, and N. Menachemi. 2017. Using structured and unstructured data to identify patients' need for services that address the social determinants of health. *International Journal of Medical Informatics* 107:101–106.

Williamson, A., J. Trott, and M. Regenstein. 2018. *Health center-based medical–legal partnerships: Where they are, how they work, and how they are funded.* National Center for Medical Legal Partnership at the George Washington University. https://medical-legalpartnership.org/wp-content/uploads/2017/12/Health-Center-based-Medical-Legal-Partnerships.pdf (accessed May 24, 2019).

7

Recommendations

In the context of a large and compelling body of evidence on how social conditions shape health, multiple factors—including the shift to value-based payment—have led to increasing experimentation with how to better integrate health care and social care services. That body of experimentation makes it clear that the health care sector is reexamining the definition of health care and how it delivers services in order to maximize individual and population health.

Better integration of health care and social care services will involve establishing the most effective and efficient roles for the health care sector to play in this area. Working from both evidence and experience, the committee recognized that enabling the health care sector to engage in activities that account for social risks and strengthen social care and community resources will require new approaches to system design, including relationships between the health and social service sectors; staffing; information and technology systems; financing; and research. Importantly, a one-size-fits-all approach is neither feasible nor advisable. The five complementary types of activities outlined by the committee in Chapter 2 to facilitate integration of social and health care—awareness, adjustment, assistance, alignment, and advocacy—are not mutually exclusive, and one does not necessarily build on another (with the exception being awareness activities, which typically are foundational to the others).

The committee drew from its evidence review and findings, presented in Chapters 2–6, to identify five goals whose accomplishment may result in better integration of social care into health care delivery, which may in turn lead to improved health and reduced health disparities. This integration includes a range of activities, including primary prevention and treatment of acute and chronic illness. The goals are to

1. Design health care delivery to integrate social care into health care, guided by the five health care system activities—awareness, adjustment, assistance, alignment, and advocacy.
2. Build a workforce to integrate social care into health care delivery.
3. Develop a digital infrastructure that is interoperable between health care and social care organizations.
4. Finance the integration of health care and social care.
5. Fund, conduct, and translate research and evaluation on the effectiveness and implementation of social care practices in health care settings.

For each goal, the committee makes actionable recommendations to provide guidance on how to achieve the goal. The goals are aimed at several audiences, including health care and social care workers, health care delivery organizations, health plans, federal and state governmental bodies, educational institutions, professional associations, foundations, and researchers.

Goal 1. Design health care delivery to integrate social care into health care.

Recommendation 1. Health care organizations should take steps to integrate social care into health care. Specific steps include

a. Make and communicate an organizational commitment to addressing health-related social needs and health disparities at the community and individual levels.
b. Recognize that comprehensive health care should include understanding an individual's social context. Evidence is rapidly accumulating concerning the most effective strategies for screening and assessing for social risk factors and social needs. Such strategies should include standardized and validated questions, as available, and should use interoperable data systems to document results.
c. Use patient-centered care models to more routinely incorporate social risk data into care decisions.
d. Design and implement integrated care systems using approaches that engage patients, community partners, frontline staff, social care workers, and clinicians in planning and evaluation and that incorporate the preferences of patients and communities.

e. Include social care workers as being integral to a team-based approach to designing and delivering health care.
f. Establish linkages and communication pathways between health care and social service providers. This is important for personal care aides, home care aides, and others who provide care and support for seriously ill and disabled patients and who have extensive knowledge of patients' social needs.
g. Develop and finance referral relationships with selected social care providers when feasible, supported by operational integration such as co-location or patient information systems. Social care providers and health care providers should establish a formal understanding and accountability within their contracting and referral relationships.
h. Support the development of those infrastructure components needed to meet the goal of care integration, including the redesign and refinement of workflows, technical assistance and support, staff with the ability to support the redesign, champions of the redesign, information on best practices, health information technology to enhance integration, and support for community partners and their infrastructure needs.

Goal 2. Build a workforce to integrate social care into health care delivery.

Recommendation 2a. State legislatures, licensing boards, professional associations, and federal agencies should develop, expand, and standardize the scopes of practice of social workers, community health workers, gerontologists, and other social care workers.

Recommendation 2b. Social workers and other social care workers[1] should be considered to be providers who are eligible for reimbursement by payers. Public and private payers should create standards for the reimbursement of social care, including assessment and such treatment as chronic care management, behavioral health integration, and transitional care management. Medicare/Medicaid payment advisory commissions should evaluate models in which social workers and other social care workers are reimbursement-eligible providers of social care services.

---

[1] In addition to social workers, the social care workforce includes nurses; physicians; community health workers; social service navigators, aides, assistants, and trained volunteers; home health aides; personal care aides; family caregivers; case managers; gerontologists; lawyers; and others.

Recommendation 2c. Funders of health care workforce training (e.g., the U.S. Department of Health and Human Services, the U.S. Department of Veterans Affairs, and foundations) should include the social care workforce in their education, training, and practice initiatives.

Recommendation 2d. Schools for health professions (including schools of medicine and nursing) as well as continuing education programs should incorporate competency-based curricula on social care. Curricula should include evidence on the social determinants of health, protocols for working in interprofessional teams to address social needs in health care settings, interpersonal and organizational approaches to advancing health equity and decreasing health disparities, and competencies relating to collecting, securing, and using data and technology to facilitate social and health care integration. Schools of health professions should also engage social workers in instructional roles in order to model their participation in interprofessional teams and to provide information on social risk screening and social care resources and referrals.

Recommendation 2e. Credentialing organizations for medicine, nursing, and other health professions should incorporate knowledge about the social determinants of health and the importance of addressing social needs in licensing examinations and continuing education requirements.

Recommendation 2f. Schools of social work as well as continuing education programs should use competency-based curricula on social care. In addition to educating students about the social determinants of health and health disparities, the curricula should include information about effective models that integrate social care and health care delivery, the interprofessional workforce, technology, and payment models that facilitate implementation and competencies relating to collecting, securing, and using data and technology to facilitate social and health care integration.

Recommendation 2g. State agencies and academic institutions, including community colleges, should develop standards for training and advancement (e.g., career ladder programs) for community health workers and other emerging social care workers.

Recommendation 2h. Foundations and other funders should commission a follow-up comprehensive report on the role of social work in health care as social care and health care integration continues to evolve.

Recommendation 2i. Foundations and other funders should fund a campaign to raise awareness among the health care professions and others about the value and contributions of social workers and other social care workers in health care.

Goal 3. Develop a digital infrastructure that is interoperable between health care and social care organizations.

Recommendation 3a. The federal government should establish a 21st-century social care digital infrastructure on a scale similar to that described in the Health Information and Technology for Economic and Clinical Health Act of 2009,[2] and it should identify and deploy policies and resources to build the internal capacity necessary for social care organizations and consumers to interoperate and interact with each other and the health care system.

Recommendation 3b. The Office of the National Coordinator should be resourced to act on the Patient Protection and Affordable Care Act of 2010[3] Section 1561 recommendations, including the adoption of modern, secure, interoperable digital systems and processes that will allow all partners to share the administrative and other data necessary to enable consumers to seamlessly obtain and maintain the full range of available health care and social care services.

Recommendation 3c. The Office of the National Coordinator should support states and regions as they identify the appropriate interoperable platforms for their communities, based on open standards and a modern technical architecture that supports flexible interfaces to allow the health and social care systems and consumers to share the structured data necessary for care coordination, avoidance of error, and a reduced burden on organizations and people being served.

Recommendation 3d. The Federal Health Information Technology Coordinating Committee should facilitate data sharing at the community level across diverse domains such as health care, housing, and education so as to support social care and health care integration.

Recommendation 3e. Integrating social care and health care requires the sharing of new types of data between new partners, some of whom are covered by the privacy rule promulgated by the Health Insurance Portability and Accountability Act of 1996[4] and some of whom are not;

[2] Public Law 111-5, February 17, 2009.
[3] Public Law 111-148, March 23, 2010.
[4] Public Law 104-191, August 21, 1996.

therefore, the U.S. Department of Health and Human Services should work with the private sector to disseminate educational tools and guidance on the data security and privacy issues that arise when collecting and sharing personally identifiable information.

Recommendation 3f. The parts of the public and private sectors involved in developing and implementing analytic and technology resources, including cell and Internet access, should do so with an explicit focus on equity; the goal should be to avoid unintended consequences such as perpetuation or aggravation of discrimination and bias and the further marginalization of populations and to proceed with an appreciation of the impact on the existing social care system.

Goal 4. Finance the integration of health care and social care.

Recommendation 4a. The Centers for Medicare & Medicaid Services should clearly define which aspects of social care that Medicaid can pay for as covered services (e.g., in the context of providing care management, targeted case management, and home- and community-based long-term care services and supports as well as within the context of managed care).

Recommendation 4b. State Medicaid agencies should use the flexibility described by the U.S. Centers for Medicare & Medicaid Services in the social care that Medicaid pays for as a covered service and make the opportunities and limitations associated with that flexibility clear to health plans and health care and social care service providers.

Recommendation 4c. The Centers for Medicare & Medicaid Services (CMS) should accelerate learning about how the integration of health and social care can improve health and reduce health care costs by encouraging and approving waivers that support social care. Sustainable financing for effective interventions piloted in the waiver should be identified by the state and CMS as an outcome of the waiver.

Recommendation 4d. States should pursue policies of continuous program eligibility to, among other benefits, create stable pools of populations for which entities can be held accountable.

Recommendation 4e. The Centers for Medicare & Medicaid Services should consider additional Medicare reforms that can broaden Medicare coverage rules in a way that is consistent with lessons from Medicaid populations and the Creating High-Quality Results and Outcomes Necessary to Improve Chronic Care Act of 2018 (the CHRONIC Care Act).[5] Health plans should take full advantage of the flexibility provided under the CHRONIC Care Act for supplemental benefits under Medicare.

Recommendation 4f. The Centers for Medicare & Medicaid Services and the states should coordinate the coverage and benefits administration of their Medicare and Medicaid dually eligible populations consistent with the emerging lessons of the financial alignment demonstrations. Efforts to improve alignment should be aggressively pursued over the short and long term, with an intentional focus on social care integration.

Recommendation 4g. The Centers for Medicare & Medicaid Services should develop incentives for health care organizations and the managed care programs that contract with Medicaid and Medicare to collaborate with community-based social services, such as area agencies on aging and centers for independent living.

Recommendation 4h. The Centers for Medicare & Medicaid Services, state Medicaid agencies, employers, and health plans should accelerate the movement to alternative payment models. The measurements aimed at assessing value in these models should include activity-based measures for social care integration and outcome measures that reflect social risk and protective factors. These value-based payment and outcome measurement models should incorporate social risk adjustment and stratification in a way that is consistent with previous recommendations (NASEM, 2016).

Recommendation 4i. The U.S. Department of Health and Human Services, payers, and other private organizations, such as foundations and institutions with community-benefit obligations, should provide funding and technical assistance to support formal contractual relationships between community-based organizations and health care entities.

Recommendation 4j. Federal and state policy makers, health plans, health systems, and private-sector investors should consider collective financing mechanisms to spread risk and create shared returns on investments in social care so that returns do not accrue to a single investor.

Recommendation 4k. Health systems subject to community benefit regulations should comply with those regulations by considering partnering

---

[5] Public Law 115-123, February 9, 2018.

with community organizations to respond to identified community gaps in social care.

Recommendation 4l. States should pursue opportunities to align their hospital licensing requirements and public reporting with federal regulations regarding community benefits to ensure consistent obligations for health systems and to explicitly link their community benefits to the provision of social care.

Goal 5. Fund, conduct, and translate research and evaluation on the effectiveness and implementation of social care practices in health care settings.

Recommendation 5a. Federal and state agencies, payers, providers, delivery systems, and foundations should contribute to advancing research on and the evaluation of the effectiveness and implementation of social care practices.

- The National Institutes of Health (NIH), the Agency for Healthcare Research and Quality (AHRQ), the Centers for Medicare & Medicaid Services (CMS), the Patient-Centered Outcomes Research Institute, the Health Resources and Services Administration (HRSA), and other funders of research and program evaluation should encourage payers, providers, and delivery systems to incorporate a range of study designs and methods that include rapid learning cycles and experimental trials.
- NIH, AHRQ, CMS, foundations, and other funders of research and program evaluation should cultivate and support researchers who have expertise in health services, social sciences, and cross-disciplinary research.
- CMS should fully finance (without state contributions) independent state waiver evaluations to ensure robust evaluation of social care and health care integration pilot programs and to facilitate the dissemination of findings.
- The U.S. Department of Health and Human Services should establish and support a clearinghouse containing information on the best and most promising practices for social care integration in order to provide "lessons learned" to health systems, community-based organizations, researchers, and others.

Recommendation 5b. Funders of health care workforce research (e.g., the Agency for Healthcare Research and Quality and foundations) should include the social care workforce in studies of the effect of the social care workforce on the health and financial outcomes of health care delivery organizations.

Recommendation 5c. The Health Resources and Services Administration and other funders should support studies of the contribution of the social care workforce, including additional workers such as gerontologists and public interest lawyers, to addressing the social determinants of health in health and community care settings.

Recommendation 5d. The Centers for Medicare & Medicaid Services, the U.S. Department of Health and Human Services, state Medicaid agencies, the National Quality Forum, and the National Committee for Quality Assurance should establish mechanisms that ensure that research on effective demonstrations informs more permanent health care reforms, including the development of accountability measures and payment models.

Recommendation 5e. To enable comparative research and evaluation, researchers, evaluators, and agencies that develop measures and standards (e.g., the National Quality Forum, the National Committee for Quality Assurance, and the Centers for Medicare & Medicaid Services) should develop a consensus on and use a common core of measures reflecting social risk and protective factors as well as key health and social outcome measures. These measures should not be limited to clinical or economic metrics, but should include patient-reported outcomes and other outcomes relevant to a range of stakeholders, including patients, families, caregivers, communities, social care organizations, health care organizations, and payers. The Agency for Healthcare Research and Quality should curate these measures in a publicly available item bank.

REFERENCE

NASEM (National Academies of Sciences, Engineering, and Medicine). 2016. *Accounting for social risk factors in Medicare payment: Criteria, factors, and methods.* Washington, DC: The National Academies Press.

Appendix

Social Need Screening Tools Comparison Table

TABLE A-1
Social Need Screening Tools Comparison Table

	AHC-Tool	HealthBegins	Health Leads
Number of social needs questions	19	24	10
Number of non-social needs questions	8	4	0
Patient or clinic population	Medicare and Medicaid	Non-specific	Non-specific
Reading level	8th grade	11th grade	6th grade
Reported completion time	NR	NR	NR
Additional languages			
Scoring	Y	Y	N
Cost	Free	Free	Free
Benefits[a]			
Caregiver responsibilities[a]			
Child care access and affordability[a]			1
Civic engagement[a]		1	
Clothing[a]			
Disabilities[a]	2		
Education[a]	1	3	
Employment[a]	1	1	
Financial strain[a]	1	2	
Food insecurity[a]	2	1	1
Health care/medicine access and affordability[a]			1
Housing insecurity/ instability/homelessness[a]	1	2	1
Housing quality[a]	1	1	
Immigration/migrant status/refugee status[a]		1	
Incarceration[a]			
Income[a]			
Interpersonal violence[a]	4	4	
Literacy[a]			1
Neighborhood safety[a]		1	
Power of attorney/guardianship[a]			
Social support[a]	2	5	1

	MLP IHELLP	Medicare Total Health Assessment Questionnaire	NAM Domains	PRAPARE	WellRx	Your Current Life Situation
	10	9	12	17	10	19
	0	30	12	4	1	10
	Non-specific	Medicare beneficiaries	Non-specific	Community health centers	Primary care	Non-specific
	8th grade	College	6th grade	8th grade	2nd grade	9th grade
	NR	10–20 min	NR	NR	NR	NR
				Spanish	Spanish	
	N	N	N	N	N	N
	Free	Free	Free	Free	Free	Free
	1					
						1
				1	1	1
				1		
	1		2	1	1	
	1			1	2	
			1			1
		2		1	1	3
				2		2
	2	1		2	1	2
	1	1				1
	2			2		
				1		
	3		1[b]	1		
	3		4	1	2	3
						1
				1	1	1
	1	1				
		2	4	1		5

continued

TABLE A-1
Continued

	AHC-Tool	HealthBegins	Health Leads
Stress[a]	1	1	
Transportation[a]	1	1	1
Utilities[a]	1		1
Veteran status[a]			
Health behaviors/behavioral health/ health status	MH, PA, SU	DP, PA	
Desire for assistance/urgent needs	Integrated into some domains; see domain-specific questions	Integrated into "civic engagement"; see domain-specific question	2 stand-alone questions

NOTE: AA = alcohol abuse; AHC = Accountable Health Community; DP = dietary pattern; HS = health/functional status; MH = mental health (including depression); MLP IHELLP = Medical-Legal Partnership Patient Screening Tool; NAM = National Academy of Medicine; NR = not reported; PA = physical activity; PRAPARE = Protocol for Responding to and Assessing Patients' Assets, Risks and Experiences; SA = substance abuse; SU = substance use; TU = tobacco use.

[a] Number refers to number of screening questions about the specified social need.

[b] Geocoded.

SOURCE: UCSF (University of California, San Francisco). *SIREN: Social Interventions Research and Evaluation Network*. 2019. https://sirenetwork.ucsf.edu (accessed April 4, 2019). Used with permission from Laura Gottlieb and Caroline Fichtenberg.

REFERENCES

Baer, T. E., E. A. Scherer, E W. Fleegler, and A. Hassan. 2015. Food insecurity and the burden of health-related social problems in an urban youth population. *Journal of Adolescent Health* 57(6):601–607.

Gundersen, C., E. E. Engelhard, A. S. Crumbaugh, and H. K. Seligman. 2017. Brief assessment of food insecurity accurately identifies high-risk U.S. adults. *Public Health and Nutrition* 20(8):1367–1371.

Hager, E. R., A. M. Quigg, M. M. Black, S. M. Coleman, T. Heeren, R. Rose-Jacobs, J. T. Cook, S. A. Ettinger de Cuba, P. H. Casey, M. Chilton, D. B. Cutts, A. F. Meyers, and D. A. Frank. 2010. Development and validity of a 2-item screen to identify families at risk for food insecurity. *Pediatrics* 126(1):e26–e32.

IOM (Institute of Medicine). 2014. *Capturing social and behavioral domains and measures in electronic health records: Phase 2*. Washington, DC: The National Academies Press.

	MLP IHELLP	Medicare Total Health Assessment Questionnaire	NAM Domains	PRAPARE	WellRx	Your Current Life Situation
		2	1	1		2
				1	1	2
				2	1	1
				1		
		AA, DP, HS, MH, PA, TU	AA, MH, PA, TU		AA, SA	
	Integrated into "immigration"; see domain-specific question	1 stand-alone question			Integrated into some domains; see domain-specific questions	2 stand-alone questions